GUTBUSTER

The
GUTBUSTER

waist loss guide

2nd edition

Garry Egger
and
Rosemary Stanton

Cartoons by Sue Plater

For men with the gut to give it a go!

ALLEN & UNWIN

Cartoons: Sue Plater
Figures: Anna Warren

First edition 1992
Reprinted 1993 (twice), 1994 (twice), 1995 (twice), 1996, 1997, 1998
Second edition 1998

Allen & Unwin
9 Atchison Street
St Leonards NSW 1590
Australia
Phone: (61 2) 8425 0100
Fax: (61 2) 9906 2218
E-mail: frontdesk@allen-unwin.com.au
Web: http://www.allen-unwin.com.au

National Library of Australia
Cataloguing-in-Publication entry:

Egger, Garry.
    The gutbuster waist loss guide: for men with
    the gut to give it a go!

    2nd ed.
    ISBN 1 86448 883 2.

    1. Weight loss. I. Stanton, Rosemary. II. Title.

613.70449

Set in 11/14pt Souvenir by DOCUPRO, Sydney
Printed and bound by Australian Print Group, Maryborough, Victoria

10 9 8 7 6 5 4 3 2 1

Contents

Introduction to the second edition

Since we wrote the first *GutBuster Waist Loss Guide* in 1992, there have been a lot of new scientific findings in the fields of obesity and weight control. We now know, for example, that there are some specific genes which, if faulty, can make it easier for some people to gain weight and more difficult for them to lose it.

Scientists have been able to breed mice that are obese—called the *ob/ob* mice. These mice have a defective *ob* gene. Normally this gene produces a hormone called leptin which regulates the level of body fat by turning off appetite. When obese mice are injected with leptin, they eat less, exercise more and lose weight. In 1994, Dr Jeffrey Feldman cloned the *ob* protein that produces leptin. This was hailed as a major breakthrough and led to great optimism that we might soon have a drug to help get rid of weight problems. Many scientists hoped that treatment of obesity might be as simple as giving people extra leptin.

However, the situation turned out to be more complicated in humans. The fatter people are, the more leptin they produce and, unlike the genetically obese mice who don't produce enough leptin, obese people produce up to four times as much as lean people. Giving them more leptin is not the answer, because they actually have some resistance to the action of leptin. Leptin doesn't turn off their appetites and stop obese people eating. The real situation now appears to be much more complicated than anybody thought.

Many obese people say that they don't ever feel hungry, in the sense of having hunger pangs. It may be that the large quantities of leptin they produce are suppressing true hunger pangs and they now eat in response to other stimuli. Whatever the genetic defects turn out to be, the major problem is that the normal controls that tell us to eat when we are hungry, and stop when we've had enough, are not working properly.

It was also thought that fat people don't actually eat too much, or indulge in too much of the wrong food, and there must be another reason why some people get as fat as pigs on a strawberry diet while others stay like racing greyhounds while eating the equivalent of two or three bullocks a day. This belief shows the inadequacy of some scientific research. There's a major problem working out what people eat, for a start. The usual method is to use a questionnaire asking what and how much someone ate on the previous day, or how much of different types of food they usually eat. From these studies it appears that fat people eat less than others. Of course, this is reinforced by the observation that when some people get fat, they eat less in front of other people—possibly because they're self-conscious or always trying to lose weight. New research technology, developed in the 1990s, makes it possible to assess accurately whether food intake matches the energy used for metabolism and exercise. By following the path through the body of a glass of water which contains harmless radioactive particles, researchers found that the average person under-estimates how much he or she eats by around 30 to 40 per cent and an obese person may under-estimate his or her intake by up to 75 per cent! There's no point in calculating how much some people *say* they eat, because they don't know. It's not that they lie, but because they seem to have an 'eye–mouth gap'—the *eye* doesn't always *see* what the hand is putting in the mouth. So some fat people may eat more than they think and they may well eat more than lean people. There are no simple answers to explain fatness without having a good look at food and exercise. Again, it's back to the drawing board.

On the exercise side of the energy equation, things have also been happening. Early exercise research concentrating on fitness suggested that you need to exercise vigorously to lose weight and get any cardio-vascular (heart) benefits. But a reanalysis in the United States Surgeon-General's Report on exercise in 1996 found that this research was based on the wrong premise. Vigorous exercise is certainly necessary for improved cardiovascular fitness, and if you are compet-ing in a sporting event, or want to improve your performance at a high level, you'll need to train hard. But any energy use involves 'burning up' calories, and the intensity of the movement is less important than how long you continue with it. Health gains, such as lower blood pressure and reduced cholesterol levels, can also come from light- to moderate-intensity movement, so vigorous gut-busting activity isn't needed here. Another return to the drawing board!

A last development we'll mention here (though it's certainly not the last to have occurred since we wrote the first edition) confirms the differences in weight gain and loss between men and women. As we pointed out previously, women store fat in different parts of the body from men, often finding it easier to gain weight and harder to lose it, both psychologically and physically. Research is now showing some reasons for this. Women may have higher levels of leptin than men, and those who exercise have an even greater leptin response following the exercise. Women, it seems, are pre-designed by nature to carry a certain level of fat and any attempts to thwart this are met by the full force of Mother Nature. Women are also influenced psychologically by pressures to conform to an idealistic body image. As a result, they are in a double bind: society tells them to diet, but their brain tells them to eat heartily. The result is often guilt and depression. Most men are less complicated and their problems come from simple ignorance. They don't know much about food or the best way to 'burn' fat. So the typical weight loss program (which is usually designed for women) is unlikely to be suitable for men.

Despite all the new and interesting findings, the drawing board is still bare. There has never been a simple answer to the problem of a pot-belly, but there are lots of ways men can help the situation. And it isn't as hard as some people think. There are plenty of short-cuts based on scientific research. We had access to what was current at the time of the first edition, and we have again searched the literature for new findings for this edition. The GutBuster program, which accompanies the book, has also grown from a small experimental program in Australia to one of the largest men's weight control programs in the world. Its results have been reported widely in scientific and clinical literature. The basic message is the same in the two editions, but there are lots of new tips and ideas in this one. Basically, what's needed are some lifestyle changes that are simple and will make life more enjoyable. There will almost certainly be even more of these discovered in the future, but for the moment we're confident that our no-nonsense, scientifically based approach to abdominal fat loss is the best option.

Introduction to the first edition

This is a different kind of 'weight control' book, for a number of reasons.

Firstly, it's aimed at men. Secondly, it's aimed at men with a very specific weight problem—a 'pot-belly' (sometimes, although incorrectly, called a 'beer gut'). This is a problem not only because it's 'unsexy', but because it's a major health hazard. Weight problems in other parts of the body are generally less of a health risk.

The major feature of this book, however, is that it concentrates on how to get rid of a 'pot-belly'. You won't have seen or heard of some of these proposed methods in any other weight control program. They include:

- throwing away your scales
- eating more often, rather than less often
- drinking alcohol if you like—but balancing it with 'trade-offs'
- forgetting about sit-ups

- moving more, but not doing any exercise you don't like
- drinking coffee (in moderation)
- eating more spicy foods
- not trying to stay excessively warm all the time
- *never* missing breakfast
- eating more!—particularly bread, cereals, fruits and vegetables
- using blankets instead of continental quilts or electric blankets.

As you read through the first part of the book, you might also be surprised to find out that:

- a 'pot-belly' could be more dangerous to your health than high cholesterol or high blood pressure
- fat on the belly is different from other fat—more dangerous, but easier to shift
- men can usually lose weight more easily than women
- it is not *how much* you eat, but *what* you eat that makes you fat
- dieting, fasting and missing meals can make you fat
- exercising before breakfast can help you lose more fat
- it's not a 'beer' gut, but a 'beer *and* peanuts' or a 'beer *and* chips' gut
- fat is often inherited.

Most of the recommendations you'll find here are based on scientific information—some are new and not yet part of 'mainstream' weight control. Where advice is based on our cumulative experience rather

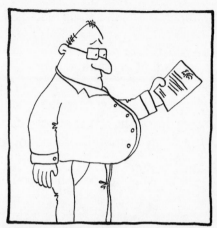

GRAHAM WERTHEIMER UPON RECEIVING
A DEMAND FROM LOCAL COUNCIL THAT
HE DEMOLISH THE UNLAWFULLY CONSTRUCTED
PATIO ABOVE THE PLAYGROUND.

than proven scientific fact, we'll tell you, offer the reasons why we suggest it and leave the decision up to you.

GutBusters was designed for men with a 'pot-belly'—who may also like a drink. This book, which goes with the program, is divided into two sections: the first (Part I) looks at some of the theory behind the program. You'll see from this why most traditional weight control programs don't work, and why weight control for men is quite different from that for women.

If you can't wait to do something about your problem, the practical side of the program is covered in Part II. You can skip straight to this and come back to Part I later. The GutBuster plan outlined in Part II is based on simple, scientific logic and has five main themes:

1 *Changing habits* that encourage over-eating and lack of exercise
2 *Eating differently*, but not necessarily *eating less*
3 *Moving more*, throughout the whole day
4 *Trading off* a limited amount of alcohol for exercise and fatty foods
5 *Plateauing*—and what to do when you stop losing weight.

The program also emphasises individual differences. The key is in understanding *your* fat problem and acting accordingly. A simple physiological explanation of how and why we gain and lose fat is also included in Appendix 1.

Before you take on the GutBuster program, test yourself for motivation on the test opposite. If you're really not motivated, you probably should forget the whole thing at this stage and come back when you are.

As we've said, the GutBuster program is unique. It started in 1991 as a program developed with the Department of Health in New South Wales, Australia. Since that time, thousands of men have successfully lost their guts and gone on to smaller and better things. The program is now accepted by obesity experts throughout the world. Results have been published in the international scientific literature and presented at scientific congresses. It's a well-backed, no-fads no-gimmicks program. And that's what we think men need

How motivated are you?

You can lead a horse to water . . . This old saying is also true of fat loss. If you're not motivated to do it, it won't happen. To score yourself on motivation, try yourself on this little test.

1 Compared with previous attempts, how motivated are you this time to lose fat?

1	2	3	4	5
Not at all motivated				Extremely motivated

2 How certain are you that you'll stay committed to a fat loss program for the time it will take to reach your goal?

1	2	3	4	5
Not at all certain				Extremely certain

3 Considering all outside factors at this time in your life—the stress you're feeling at work, your family obligations, etc.—to what extent can you tolerate the effort required to stick to a healthy eating plan?

1	2	3	4	5
Cannot tolerate				Can tolerate easily

4 Think honestly about how much weight you hope to lose and how quickly you hope to lose it. Figuring a weight loss of 0.5–1 kilogram per week, how realistic is your expectation?

1	2	3	4	5
Very unrealistic				Very realistic

---

5   While dieting, do you fantasise about eating a lot of your favourite foods?

1	2	3	4	5
Always	Frequently	Occasionally	Rarely	Never

6   How confident are you that you can work regular exercise into your daily schedule, starting tomorrow?

1	2	3	4	5
Not at all confident				Extremely confident

Your score:

6–12:   You're not very serious about this. Come back when you are!

13–24: You're reasonably motivated. But you may need some help.

25+:   Your motivation is high. Let's get to it.

---

in this age of hype and unsupported pseudo-scientific sounding promises. We're sure you'll see the sense of the GutBuster program and start feeling its benefits, even after the first week. We've set a goal for you to lose 1 per cent of your gut a week—at least over the first couple of months—and that amount of weight loss should quickly become obvious as well as feel good.

Part I

Why a pot-belly is a health hazard

1 Why a special weight loss plan for men?

Men and women *are* different. Not just in the obvious ways, but also in some less obvious ones. For example, there are differences in where and why men and women get fat. Women—at least in their reproductive years—tend to store fat around the hips and buttocks. Men store it around the waist—hence the male 'pot-belly' or 'beer gut'.

We're now beginning to understand the reasons for this, but we don't have all the answers. However, it's likely that male fat has developed in response to the need for quick energy—a legacy from the days when man was the hunter. Female fat is needed more as an energy store for reproduction. From Mother Nature's point of view, it's important for women to have energy reserves so they can survive the nine months of pregnancy, even if food is scarce, to progenerate the human species. Men are only important for a few minutes (sometimes less!). On the swings and roundabouts principle, though, our big payback comes later in life when Mother Nature deserts the female of the species after menopause, but still allows us our couple of minutes of sunshine, right into our twilight years!

It *is* known that:

- More than one in two men in industrialised countries have 'pot-bellies' which could put them at increased risk of serious health problems
- as many as three in four men among blue-collar workers and older men have a 'pot-belly' which could potentially kill them
- fat stored on the abdomen as a 'pot-belly' is a risk factor for heart disease, diabetes, high blood pressure and other health problems. It can also cause snoring, bad back, bad knees and impotence
- men with a family history of heart disease or diabetes significantly increase their personal risk by carrying fat around the gut
- most men can lose their 'pot-belly' with relative ease—if they go about it the right way.

More than one in two men in industrialised countries have a 'pot-belly' which could potentially kill them.

Until recently, most weight loss programs concentrated on methods that would appeal to women. Neither men nor women have seen the male 'gut' as a health problem and few people have tried to persuade men that they should get rid of it. There's been no real pressure to want to do anything about it. Both men and women have thought that men who may not *look* fat other than around the middle of their bodies had no need for urgent action. Hence, almost every diet book has tried to appeal mainly to women. *The GutBuster plan is especially for men!*

The fattening of the industrialised world

Men have typically chosen to think of themselves as tough and resilient. Indeed, this image was probably fair in the early pioneering years and perhaps through to the middle of this century. Old war pictures, family camping photos and even old movies show that men in those days rarely had a belly. Could you imagine the Lone Ranger carving up the country with his belly hanging over Silver's neck?

In the early days, life was tough. Most men and women worked hard for a feed and, when it came, the energy taken in was quickly used up working for the next one. But by the 1960s, the advanced countries of the world faced some enormous changes in the way they found food and the activity they undertook. It was no longer necessary for most people to work hard physically to make a living. There was more sedentary work coupled with more sedentary leisure. At the same time, there was a huge expansion in the food supply. Supermarkets expanded the number of foods available from around 600 to more than 10 000 different food items. In some countries, even more foods are now available. Food was not only plentiful but high in fat—a nutrient which, until recent times in evolution, was relatively hard to come by. And as we know, you can eat less food in volume but take in more fat and end up getting fatter.

There had always been a few fat people, but these changes meant that more people in the industrialised world started to get fat. They also smoked more, ate more fatty foods and experienced the effects of unrelieved stress. As a result of these changes, deaths from heart disease in many countries reached new heights in the late 1960s.

In the years following, better-educated people became aware of some of the risk factors. Many gave up smoking and the number of men smoking continues to decrease. Some people made jogging and then aerobics and weight training, a way of life. They attended stress management courses, went to gyms, ate 'healthy' food and generally took better care of themselves.

As a result, the pattern of health of men in many countries changed. Instead of the working man being healthy and the executive unhealthy, the reverse occurred. Even so, across all stratas of society, men in general have lagged well behind women in their indices of health and well-being. Even with all the advances in health treatments, men's life expectancy still averages seven years less than that of women, and men suffer more heart disease, cancers (except for breast cancer), diabetes, injury and deaths from violence.

From the late 1970s, the working man was especially at risk. As machines started to take over the workplace, physical work gave way to operating machinery. Body fat in men that was once kept at bay through daily work now accumulates while they sit on forklifts or cranes or drive vehicles that do most of the heavy physical work. The increased use of computers,

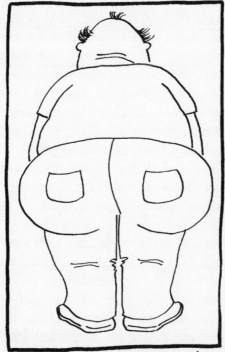

MILTON BARGEASSE WAS SO BIG HE
NEEDED A BRAIN IN EACH BUTTOCK
TO CONTROL HIS *LOWER BODY.*

and the decrease in activity from long periods spent sitting in front of them, has exacerbated the problem. The computer industry is probably the biggest potential customer of the weight control industry.

How fat are we? According to the latest figures from the United States, the United Kingdom and Australasia, we are very fat. Surveys show that around 50 to 60 per cent of men and 30 to 40 per cent of women are overweight or obese. In some groups of American

Indians, Australian Aborigines and African-American women, the figures are even higher. Various surveys of schoolchildren have also shown that the incidence of obesity in children has doubled in the last 20 years. For the first time, non-insulin dependent diabetes (NIDDM), sometimes called 'late onset' diabetes because it usually occurs later in life, is being seen in adolescents. Non-insulin dependent diabetes is strongly associated with obesity, particularly abdominal obesity.

So the myths of the tough American cowboy, the bronzed Aussie surfer and the wiry English explorer are dead. Today we're faced with a portly generation of fat, unfit, pot-bellied men who would get tired *flying* over the North-West Trail—let alone walking it!

In women, the trend to increasing fatness may have been hidden by clothing manufacturers. The average woman's dress size, for example, has increased a size and a half over the past 20 years. Cunningly, manufacturers have kept to the old sizes while increasing the measurements. So a size 12 in Australia, the average size which used to fit an 85 centimetre waist and 95 centimetre hip, is now 6 centimetres bigger in both places.

Young women often manage to stay slim—sometimes too thin for their health. It's only when women reach their forties and fifties that a significant number start to get too fat. For men, the picture is different. *They* start to get fat in their twenties and by their mid-thirties, the pot-belly is firmly in place. More than half of all men in their late thirties are overweight or obese. More women of the same age are underweight than overweight in Australia, although not in some other countries. The irony is that young women, many of whom are already thin, make the most effort to lose weight. Men tend to ignore their excess flesh.

Levels of overweight in the industrialised world*

- More than one in two men and one in three women are overweight or obese ('obesity' is defined as more than 20 per cent over ideal weight).
- This ranges from 25 per cent of 20–24-year-old men to 60 per cent of over-45-year-olds and from 17 per cent of 20–24-year-old women to 57 per cent over-65-year-old women.
- At least 25–33 per cent of under-16-year-olds are also overweight or obese.
- The level of obesity is increasing by just over 1 per cent per year.
- The average female dress size has increased a size and a half since the 1960s (i.e. a size 12 is now 6 centimetres bigger at the waist and hips).
- Average trouser waists for men have increased from 87 centimetres to 90–93 centimetres.

* Figures vary from country to country. These statistics are based on Australian figures and are generally representative.

The problems with being too fat

There are three major kinds of health problem associated with being too fat:

1 diseases such as heart disease, diabetes, gallstones, arthritis and several types of cancer

2   increased risk factors for disease such as high blood
    pressure, high blood cholesterol and high triglycer-
    ides (a type of fat in the blood)
3   less obvious problems such as back pain, sore
    knees, snoring and getting over-tired.

You may know about the first problem (although our
research shows most men are pretty vague about this),
but you may be surprised to know that having a
pot-belly can make you snore more! This is because
the tongue, as well as the belly, is one of the first parts
of a man's body to get fat. This can block the air
passage, or pharynx, during sleep, so that you sound
like a lumberjack's mate. It may also drive your bedmate
to distraction!

---

*One of the most significant causes of snoring
and obstructive sleep apnoea (OSA) is being
overweight.*

Snoring is part of a syndrome of sleeping problems
known as obstructive sleep apnoea (OSA), which is
most common amongst overweight men. Obstructive
sleep apnoea involves poor breathing at night, which
can mean that the body doesn't get the oxygen it needs
to keep you healthy. The heart may have to work
harder and this could push up blood pressure. Because
there's a real danger of dying from lack of oxygen, the
brain (one part of the body that, fortunately, is still
working) will wake you up in brief spurts to get you
breathing again. You may not be aware of it, but these
little periods of disturbed sleep that snorers snaffle and

grovel through could happen hundreds of times a night. And you wonder why you're tired during the day!

Fat men who are heavy snorers often think they're great sleepers. They say they never suffer with insomnia. And of course they don't. They suffer from the opposite—*hyper*somnia, or the need for too much sleep. Because they wake unconsciously so often during the night, they're asleep at their desks, or at the wheel of their car or truck, during the day while the body tries to make up for the disturbances at night.

Problems with being too fat		
Diseases	**Risk factors**	**Less obvious**
Heart disease	High blood pressure	Back problems
Diabetes	High cholesterol	Snoring/OSA
Gallstones	High blood sugars	Lack of energy
Osteoarthritis	Lack of fitness	Hypersomnia
Bowel cancer	High triglycerides	Knee problems
Breast cancer		Skin problems
Uterine cancer		Breathing problems
		Foot infections
		Sex problems

Backache is another problem for the fat-bellied man. The reason is fairly obvious. Try hanging a dead sheep on a stick of willow and see what happens to the willow. The trouble is that, when the human spine bends, it doesn't snap back like willow. It can pull on or pinch nerves and muscles that are designed to hold it upright. The only solution is to take the pressure off by getting rid of some of the weight.

A similar thing happens to the knees. As major joints between the gut and the ankle, they have to take a lot of the weight, especially in the flexed position when climbing stairs or walking up hills. The greater the bend in the knee, the greater the multiplication of the load it has to carry. And any self-respecting knee can only take so much.

Many people are also unaware of skin problems in fat people. Underneath the fold of fat that makes up an overhanging gut in a man, it can get hot and damp and be a breeding ground for lots of micro-organisms. Intertrigo is a type of eczema that can form under the fat layer, causing itching and rashes.

The feet also suffer. Having extra weight forcing down on the two pads responsible for keeping the body upright is a bit like what would happen to two raisins on sticks asked to hold up a pumpkin. If the feet are enclosed in 'non-breathing' leather shoes, and heavy

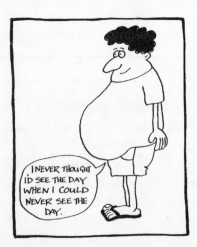

woollen socks are worn, the feet are likely to overheat and perspire. With no mechanism for cooling, this can cause rashes and skin problems on the feet.

Sex problems associated with having a pot-belly hardly bear mentioning. Suffice to say that you can't build a shed if you can't find the tools. It might be worth pointing out, though, that testosterone, the male hormone asssociated with 'friskiness', decreases with an increase in belly size. So if your bedroom athletics are suffering, it just could be your girth size that's doing it. In any case, even if it's only from your partner's point of view, getting rid of a belly is not going to be a disadvantage in the horizontal dancing caper.

2 Fat: What it is and how you get it

We have learned a lot about muscle over the past 20 years, probably because of its role in sport and athletic performance. There are now exercise physiologists, sports scientists, physiotherapists and a range of other professionals whose lives are taken up with finding out how muscles work and how to make them work better. But what about fat? Have you ever heard of a 'fatologist' or a 'fat physiologist'? It's unlikely. Yet there are 'fat farms' and weight control clinics dotted around the country, all claiming to provide the truth and light about fat reduction. There are also myriad weight control books and articles in popular magazines, although few of them relate back to a true scientific, or sometimes even a logical, base.

Our knowledge of fat *has* increased over the last decade. In fact, scientists have probably found out more in that time than ever before. And what we now know shows that the topic is much more complicated than we originally thought. A simple explanation is outlined below. For those who are more interested, a detailed explanation of how fat cells function and what this means for fat loss is included in Appendix I.

Fat and fat cells

The body is made up of billions of cells in bones, skin, organs, muscle and fat. Fat cells are similar to other cells but they have a small pool or reservoir of fat, as shown in Figure 1.

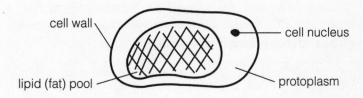

Figure 1: Fat cell

This acts as an energy store which can increase or decrease in size depending on how much energy we use up in staying alive and moving around, and how much energy we take in from what we eat and drink.

A pot-belly is nothing more than a huge mass of swollen fat cells. If you cut off all the white fatty bits on a big pile of T-bone steaks, put them in a plastic bag and tied them around your middle, you'd have a similar lump of fat. Horrible thought, isn't it?

Excess fat comes when you take in more energy from food and drinks than you use up for metabolism and exercise. But this isn't the whole story. It doesn't explain why some people get fat more easily than others, or why some get fat all over, while others get fat on the stomach or on other parts of the body. *Genetics* and *gender* also play a part.

Genes help determine your size and shape—you can inherit an ability to gain or lose fat easily. Obesity can run in families. Sometimes it runs in families who all eat and drink too much. In other cases, obesity runs in families because their genes mean they don't burn up excess energy easily.

Fat in your genes

Scientists around the world have being studying the influence of genetics on body fat and fat distribution. Their findings show the following:

- Superficial fat, or the fat just under the skin, is not influenced much by genetic effects (probably only about 5 per cent). Fat mass, or total body fat, which makes up around 25–30 per cent of body fat, is controlled by genetics. This suggests that deep fat (internal fat) may be the fat component which is inherited.
- About 45–60 per cent of all forms of fat can be transmitted from generation to generation; however, depending on the type of fat measured, this could be either through inheritance, or be due to family patterns of eating and drinking.
- Genetics can predispose someone to being fat but, unlike the eye or hair colour which you inherit, the environment of food and activity determines whether you will actually get fat.
- Genetics seems to affect the fat-free or muscle mass more than other measures of fat, but genetics

---

combined with family upbringing influences the percentage of body fat, fat mass and fat distribution.

- Neither parent independently seems to have any greater effect than the other in genetically influencing fat measures in their offspring.
- New gene discoveries have shown that one gene, called *ob*, is responsible for a hormone called leptin which is involved in suppression of appetite. Another gene, UCP_2, may help some people lose energy as heat faster than others, and therefore make it easier for them to stay lean.

If your gene pool doesn't have a shallow end, you may find it harder to slim down than someone with 'lean genes'. That doesn't mean that slimming down is impossible. Fat genes are not like the genes for fair

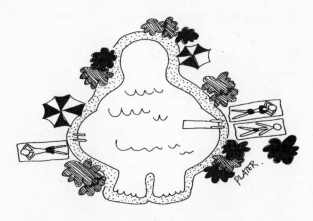

The Modern Gene Pool.

hair or blue eyes: they don't mean that being fat is inevitable. What they do imply is that, given the right circumstances—the wrong kind of food and not enough exercise—it will be easier for someone with 'fat' genes to put on fat than someone from a leaner background. So let's not kid ourselves: it may be a little more difficult if you picked the wrong parents. But remember, irrespective of your genes, we now live in an *obesogenic* environment. Everything in modern society is designed to make things easier for us. Unfortunately, in doing so, it can also make us fat.

It may not be as good as a gene test, but you can gain an idea of your genetic liabilities from the quiz shown in the box below.

Testing your genes

1 As far as you know, were either or both of your parents significantly overweight for most of their lives?

	Score
Neither/don't know	0
Yes, one parent	1
Yes, both parents	2

2 Do you have any brothers or sisters who have been significantly overweight for most of their lives?

No	0
Yes, one	1
Yes, more than one	2

---

3   When did you first become overweight?

After 20	0
During my teens	1
Before my teens	2

4   How difficult do you find it to take off weight?

Not difficult at all	0
Reasonably difficult	1
Very difficult	2

5   Where do you mainly get fat when you put on weight?

On the stomach	0
On the hips and buttocks	1
All over	2

Scores:

0–4: Your weight problem does not appear to be significantly genetically related. This means it is related to lifestyle and therefore the problem should be quite easy to solve if you are committed to doing so.

5–7: There appears to be a moderate hereditary component to your weight problem. This means you may find it a little harder to lose fat than some of your friends. You may need help from a dietitian, but your problems should not be too difficult to overcome.

8–10: There appears to be a significant hereditary component to your weight problem. This means you may need special help and closer attention from a dietitian. With the proper approach and a long-range plan, you should be able to overcome your bad start.

If your specific weight problem is a pot-belly (which is what this book is about), it's more than likely that your major problem is not inherited fat, but has more to do with your lifestyle—what you eat, drink and how you move. An imbalance in food, drink and exercise will give you the 'apple' or android shape—a bit like a pregnant telephone pole. The man who is genetically fat is usually fat all over with an ovoid shape. This problem is usually apparent from early in life.

Gender is also important: women have a higher percentage of body fat than men and it is stored in different locations on the body. Women are usually more pear-shaped (called gynoid), unless they are genetically overweight. The differences in shapes between men and women offer some reasons why women often find it harder to lose fat than men. However, because sex hormones vary in different people, there are exceptions to the body shape and gender rule. A few men are pear-shaped and a somewhat similar proportion of women are apple-shaped. After menopause, the apple shape becomes more common in women. Losing fat may be easier for these women and harder for the pear-shaped men than the more characteristic gender shapes.

Not if you're fat but where

Fat cells around the abdomen in men are different from those on the hips, buttocks and thighs of women.

Abdominal fat cells are generally smaller and more active. This means they inject fat into the bloodstream more readily when the body needs it and they also take more fat from the blood when there is more than the body needs for fuel to power the muscles. Even more dangerous are fat stores around the middle now known as visceral fat. Visceral fat is stored around the organs, such as the stomach, liver, kidneys and intestines. Visceral fat has been shown to be up to seven times more active than gluteal fat and three times more active than subcutaneous abdominal fat. This means it's released into the bloodstream even faster than other fats. A bigger problem is that visceral fat is not obvious, like a pot-belly. However it generally—although not always—correlates with abdominal fat. Like abdominal fat, it's also much easier to shift than female-type gluteal fat.

The bad news about all this is that fat-bellied men

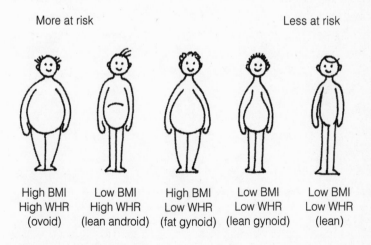

More at risk   Less at risk

High BMI	Low BMI	High BMI	Low BMI	Low BMI
High WHR	High WHR	Low WHR	Low WHR	Low WHR
(ovoid)	(lean android)	(fat gynoid)	(lean gynoid)	(lean)

BMI—body mass index   WHR—waist:hip ratio

Figure 2: Body fat distribution and health risk

can have lots of extra fat lying round in their blood-stream. This is the major reason for the increase in risk of heart disease, diabetes, gallstones, high blood cholesterol and high blood pressure. It's also responsible for the reduction in the pot-bellied man's general lack of fitness and inability to be able to . . . well, do things.

It's important to realise that you don't have to be fat all over to be at risk. In fact, as Figure 2 shows, the lean man with a gut (shaped like an apple), is more at risk than the fat man without a gut who is shaped like a pear, or even the man who is fat all over—like the box the fruit comes in!

3 Losing fat: Some ways and means

Now for some good news. Once a man makes an effort to lose fat, it usually comes off his stomach faster than it comes off other parts of the body. A *fat*-bellied man then can become a *flat*-bellied man fairly easily!

Women have more problems losing fat from some areas of their bodies. The larger fat cells on their hips, buttocks and thighs are less active and have an important role in reproduction to provide energy during pregnancy and lactation, if needed. These fat cells resist being moved. Nature put them there for the survival of the species in case of famine when the woman must provide for the needs of a baby.

But that's not all. Swedish researchers have shown that when men and women with roughly the same fat composition start on an exercise program, women tend to eat relatively more after exercise than men—without knowing it! Other research shows that this may be associated with changes in leptin levels (the hormone associated with appetite) which occur after exercise and dieting in women, but which do not occur to the same extent in men. Exercise does help women lose fat, but they lose less fat after an exercise program than men do.

For a variety of reasons, women store fat more readily and lose it less readily than men.

Women who think that starvation is the ideal way to lose fat as fast as men are also in for disappointment. Fat stores on women's hips, buttocks and thighs are more resistant to severe dieting than fat stores elsewhere on the female body or fat stored on men's bodies. Female hormones are the cause of this reduced ability for women to lose fat from the lower body. Nature likes to preserve energy stores for reproduction. Stores of fat on the hips, buttocks and thighs ensure that the pregnant or feeding mother can provide enough energy for her child. After menopause, when women no longer bear children, they store fat more around the belly and on the upper body. Their shape becomes more similar to that of men. They also develop similar health problems to men and heart disease, high blood pressure, diabetes and gallstones become more common after menopause.

The good news for younger women is that fat around the hips, buttocks and thighs has no apparent link to ill-health—apart from perhaps a slight increase in the risk of varicose veins. With gender and fat it seems that what you lose on the roundabouts you pick up on the swings!

A summary of sex differences in fat loss

In losing body fat, women differ from men in that they generally have:

- a higher proportion of body fat (15–30 per cent of body mass compared with 12–24 per cent in males)
- a greater proportion of fat stored in lower body gluteal fat cells which have greater enzyme activity and thus a higher capacity to store fat
- less lean muscle tissue and hence a lower resting metabolic rate and a lower overall need for energy
- greater resistance to fat loss in gluteal cells following food restriction
- greater compensation of energy intake following exercise
- a potentially greater appetite for high density fatty foods if they repeatedly restrict energy intake with yoyo dieting and frequent ups and downs in body weight
- more labile fat stores on the breast and upper body than on the hips and lower body.

Metabolic rate and what it means

Metabolism is what is happening in your body while your mind is making other plans. You need energy to keep you alive—to digest food, get blood to the muscles and organs, feed your brain, keep you warm and breathing. These basic functions make up metabolism and the energy to carry them out is called resting metabolic rate or RMR. It includes only the energy needed to keep you alive at rest. Energy for any physical activity is additional. The resting metabolic rate can be thought of as being like a fire, with the embers burning continually. If the fire can be stoked up, it uses more energy. If it's left to run down, it uses less.

For the average-sized person, RMR uses around one Calorie (or 4.2 kilojoules) per minute. (For the technically minded, this is 70 Watts—about the same rate of energy usage as a 75 Watt light globe.) If you consider that a standard glass of beer is the equivalent of approximately 100 Calories, this means that the average person would need around 100 minutes at rest to burn the energy in one beer. Walking briskly, on the other hand, burns between 5 and 6 Calories a minute, so you could theoretically burn up a beer with 15–20 minutes of walking (although it doesn't actually happen like this because of the body's ability to adjust to changes in energy).

The key factor in working out how many calories your body burns is RMR or metabolic rate at rest. This makes up about 70 per cent of the total energy we use in a day, so it has big implications for fat burning. If we can increase RMR—even by only around 10 per cent—it will help fat loss. Every kilogram of fat has the equivalent energy of about 7700 kilojoules (3500 Calories), so an increase in RMR of 10 per cent would mean (again, theoretically) that you could lose about 7 kilograms of fat in a year—without doing anything!

The scientific evidence that RMR can be increased by

Contributions to total energy use

Metabolic rate	70%
Movement	20%
Thermic (heat) effects	10%
–food[*]	
–fidgeting[#] etc.	

[*]   Up to 25 per cent of calories from carbohydrates are wasted by
      the thermic effect of digesting carbohydrate compared with only
      3 per cent wastage when fat is eaten. It takes a lot of energy to
      convert carbohydrates to fat.

[#]   Fidget-type activity may make up 50 per cent of the thermic
      effect of movement.

this much is a bit mixed, but there are positive signs in
several areas. Some of the ways covered below will help
your health, even if they don't help decrease your gut.
We're confident, though, that they'll also help to do that.

Exercise

Aerobic exercise is one of the most significant ways to
influence RMR. Not only does this burn up energy while
you're doing it (as we shall see later), but it may help
burn extra energy by raising RMR for up to 24 hours
afterwards. Think of the exercise as being like starting
a fire which then burns down slowly, continuing to
generate heat for some time afterwards.

The idea that ten minutes of walking burns only 60
Calories is not totally accurate. If you walk regularly,
to the point where it raises RMR by 10 per cent even
over twelve hours, walking for ten minutes could burn
an extra 72 Calories, or 132 Calories over a twelve-hour

period. Calorie charts for exercise in most diet programs do not give you a true picture, unless they
include 24-hour values. So far, these are not available.

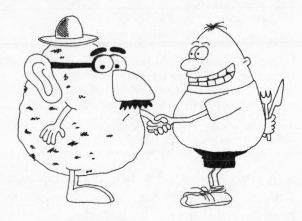

MR POTATO HEAD MEETS MR PUMPKIN BELLY

Food

If you have a fire which has died down to ashes and you
want it to burn a log, you need to get the fire going
again. In the same way, the body needs more energy
than the basal metabolic rate to digest food. In scientific
terms, this is called the thermic effect of food, or TEF.
The TEF has been shown to increase metabolic rate by
10–40 per cent for up to six hours after a meal. This
could account for up to 10 per cent of daily energy
expenditure, but will vary according to the amount and
composition of food and how often you eat.

The implications of this are quite significant. Eating

certain foods like spices might add to the TEF (as we shall see below). Even more important is the frequency and time of eating. Eating small meals more often burns more energy than eating big meals less often. *Grazing* is better than *gorging*, provided the total amount of energy consumed over the day is the same.

For some people, a grazing style of eating is not a good idea, either because every eating occasion is a time for over-eating, or because they choose foods with poor nutritional value between meals. Grazing works only when you spread out the same amount of foods, not when you eat more.

Eating breakfast is also important because breakfast gets the metabolism going. Once your body digests breakfast, it starts burning more calories. A good breakfast is likely to be burned off more effectively than a big dinner. Skipping breakfast or lunch and eating most of your day's food at the end of the day is one of the worst habits for weight loss. Eating small and often is much better, although you should read our hints about appropriate foods. Snacking on chocolates, chips or sweets throughout the day is not what we have in mind!

Eating several small meals during the day is a better way of losing fat than eating only one large meal.

Caffeine

Caffeine comes in tea, coffee and cola drinks. It's a stimulant and an addictive drug. However, used carefully, caffeine may have some advantages in weight control. (For a detailed explanation of why this may be so, refer to the explanation on fat cell function in Appendix 1.) First you need to understand some of the properties of addiction.

The symptoms of addiction are:

- craving
- withdrawal
- tolerance
- analgesia
- consciousness alteration.

Craving means you want more of the addictive substance as you get used to it. With caffeine, this can be controlled if you restrict yourself to a certain intake. Check the table below for caffeine concentrations of various foods and drinks.

Caffeine concentration of foods and drinks	
Food item	**Caffeine (mg/75 ml)**
Coffee	
Expresso, short black or flat white (150 ml)	70–90
Drip filter or percolated (150 ml)	70–80
Instant, 250 ml mug	60–90
Tea, average strength, 1 cup	25–35
Tea, weak, 1 mug, 250 ml	20
Cola, 1 can, 370 ml	35
Cola, extra strong e.g. Jolt, 1 can	50–72
Chocolate bar (small)	20–25
Cocoa, 2 teaspoons	6–8

Withdrawal refers to the symptoms you suffer if a substance to which you are addicted is not available for an extended period. Heavy coffee drinkers typically get headaches and 'the jitters' if they don't get their daily dose. The trick is not to get used to having such high quantities in the first place.

Tolerance suggests that once you become habituated to a drug, you need more of it to get the same effect from it. And here is the key to the possible benefits of caffeine in weight control. Because caffeine is a stimulant, it can have mild effects in increasing metabolic rate. Used with other techniques such as increased exercise and a grazing style of eating, a moderate daily intake of caffeine might have some metabolic benefits for those wanting to lose weight. As long as the quantity is not more than three to four cups of coffee a day, there should be few side-effects. If you drink more coffee or other caffeine-containing drinks, however, the tolerance effect means that you'll continually keep needing more to have the same effect. If you become an habitual high-dose caffeine consumer, the habituation will eliminate any benefits.

You may have noticed this before. If you drink several cups of coffee every day, it seems to have little effect on your mental state. But if you drink only one or two, each cup seems to noticeably increase mental alertness.

The effect is even greater for someone who has gone off caffeine altogether or who doesn't consume it at all. If you're currently a heavy caffeine consumer, you should go 'cold turkey' and have no caffeine at all for two weeks, then begin to drink a maximum of two cups a day (one in the morning, one in the afternoon) at the start of your GutBuster program. If you don't drink much caffeine, restrict yourself to a maximum of two cups a day. You may also take one to two cups of tea and one to two glasses of a diet cola drink if you wish, because these have lower caffeine levels. However, remember that the acidity of diet cola drinks can damage tooth enamel. Always rinse your mouth with plain water after drinking any soft drink, whether or not it contains sugar. They are all acidic.

We should mention that the effect of caffeine on RMR is likely to be much less than the effects of exercise and a grazing eating style. We should also add that the scientific evidence on caffeine and fat loss is fairly limited. Don't forget also that we're talking about caffeine. Don't think the possible fat loss effect applies to all coffees, such as coffee with cream, cappuccino or cafe latte. As we'll see, the kilojoules and fat in the milk or cream will negate any kilojoule-burning effects of the caffeine in these drinks.

Smoking and caffeine

If you are a smoker and a heavy coffee drinker, your choices are more limited. For some reason that is not yet clear, cigarette smoke seems to dampen the effects of caffeine. When you quit (which anyone with half a brain would do), blood caffeine levels rise, even though you may not be drinking more coffee. The effects of this are increased nervousness, jittery feelings and a desire to have—you guessed it—a cigarette. Hence quitting smoking should also mean quitting caffeine, at least until the withdrawal symptoms of nicotine have passed.

The problem then is that (a) if quitting smoking can lead to weight gain (which we know it can) and (b) quitting caffeine can lead to a decrease in metabolic rate, the combined effect of quitting both is likely to have a double whammy effect on your weight.

The way to get around this is to do even more of the other activities that increase metabolic rate, especially aerobic exercise.

Spicy foods

It may sound odd, but some research has shown that foods such as curries, satays or hot Thai dishes—or any food containing lots of chilli—can increase metabolic rate for a short time after a meal. This may be due to a natural ingredient in chillies called capsaicin. Research is still continuing into this, but because chilli and spices can make low-fat food taste good, there's not likely to be much harm in giving it a go. Adding some low-fat spicy dishes to your weekly meals makes eating more interesting, and might burn up more than the parts of the body that usually burn after a good curry.

There is a rider to this. Research on monosodium glutamate (MSG), an additive used to bring out the flavour in many Chinese and Japanese meals, suggests that it may be an appetite stimulant. Using rats, researchers have shown that MSG acts on a part of the brain that makes you eat more. However, against this is the fact that very few Chinese or Japanese people are overweight. Perhaps the easiest solution if you're having a Chinese meal is to ask which dishes have been prepared without MSG. Say yes to chilli, no to MSG. Also, be aware that a lot of fat can be added to some Asian-style curries in the form of coconut milk. As a highly saturated fat, this is not only fattening, but also potentially unhealthy for the heart.

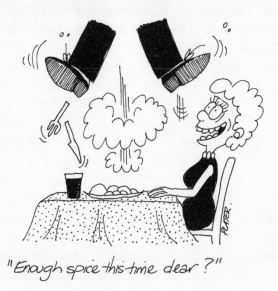

"Enough spice this time dear?"

Body temperature

Air temperature is another factor that influences metabolic rate. In cold climates, your body works harder to maintain body temperature and keep you warm and this requires energy. If the weather is cold enough to make you shiver, you'll burn even more energy. One well-known Sydney doctor used to go round his draughty hospital all winter shivering in his shirt sleeves—it was his way of keeping his weight down. In parts of the world where it is very cold, those who work outside may burn one and a half times as many calories as people in warm climates. In hot climates, on the other hand, metabolism decreases because body temperature is easily maintained.

You don't need great differences in air temperature for an effect to be apparent. Researchers have measured the metabolic rate of individuals over 24 hours at temperatures of either 20°C or 28°C. At the lower temperature, metabolic rate was an average of 5 per cent higher and in some people the difference was as high as 12 per cent. If this is translated into potential weight loss, it could theoretically mean a difference of around 100 Calories a day in the average person—or up to 5 kilograms of body fat in a year!

This makes a mockery of sauna or steam baths that you find in clubs filled to overflowing by pot-bellied men hoping to 'sweat it off'. Any *weight* loss from saunas comes from sweat, or water loss, which is quickly replaced. It's not *fat*. In theory at least, regular heat treatments like saunas could cause you to *gain* fat because they may lower metabolic rate.

To lose fat, you don't have to sit in a refrigerator, although it's probably only a matter of time until some smart operator starts selling cold rooms to the fat farms. It also doesn't mean sitting in draughts, or letting yourself get cold. But it could mean avoiding simple situations of overheating such as putting on your car heater, having central heating in your home, using electric blankets, huddling over a radiator or wearing

very heavy clothing. By allowing your body to create
its own warmth, you could help mould your middle.

Let's make it clear that there have not been any
scientific studies to show that people lose weight better
without heaters. But we do know that allowing your
body to create some of its own warmth uses up extra
calories. It also makes scientific sense, athough you're
unlikely to read about it in many weight loss programs.
And even if staying cool doesn't help your gut, it could
help your skin. Many skin specialists now claim that
common forms of overheating can be major causes of
skin problems. Their recommendations for skin health
could be just as useful for fat loss. They include:

- *Avoiding continental quilts and electric blankets*: A
  continental quilt, or doona, can be the equivalent
  of six blankets which can't be shed gradually as you
  heat up. Go for blankets, including some cotton
  blankets, even in winter.

- *Not over-dressing*: Although it's tempting to rug up
  in heavy, warm clothing in winter, you're likely to
  use up more energy if you dress lightly—even if
  you're a little cool. Men with an overhanging mound
  of flesh around the middle can also suffer skin
  problems in that part which never sees the light—or
  air. Adding heavy clothing to trap in the heat is
  likely to make it worse.

- *Avoiding heaters and airconditioning if you can*:
  Much of our life is spent in controlled environments
  which reduce the body's ability to adapt. A little
  cool is not such a bad thing.

- *Reducing foot temperature*: A lot of heat gets

trapped around the feet, especially with modern footwear and heavy woollen socks. While ventilating your feet won't dramatically alter your metabolic rate, it could help. It could also help prevent skin problems of the feet caused by excess weight bearing down on those little pinkies.

If you don't have good breathing shoes and good cotton socks, one way to increase ventilation is to punch half a dozen holes with a hole punch in the instep of your most worn shoes or boots. This might seem a bit stupid, but anybody who is down grovelling close enough to your shoes to notice is going to look even more stupid.

Testing your metabolism

Metabolic rate can be tested accurately in a number of ways. The most common uses the same technique that accurately measures cardiovascular fitness in a laboratory. With a sophisticated gas analysis machine, an experienced tester can measure the amount of oxygen you inhale and the carbon dioxide you exhale every minute you're connected to the machine. From this, a formula is used to work out your oxygen consumption per kilogram of body weight per minute. This is a reflection of the amount of energy your body is burning at rest to keep you alive.

Nowhere near as sophisticated is our own little test of metabolism shown in the table below. Try this to get at least a rough idea of whether your metabolism is weighing you down as much as your belly.

Testing your metabolism

1 Do you currently participate in any regular activity or program, either on your own or in a formal class, designed to improve your fitness or keep your weight down?

   1 Never
   2 Rarely
   3 Occasionally
   4 Often (e.g. more than three times a week)

2 In the past twelve months, have you crash dieted or fasted at any stage (i.e. for more than a day)?

   1 Yes, several times
   2 Yes, once or twice
   3 No

3 Do you eat breakfast

   1 Rarely or never
   2 Occasionally
   3 Often or always?

4 Do you always try to avoid being even mildly cold in winter?

   1 Yes
   2 Not really

5 How many cups of coffee/tea do you drink in an average day?

   1 None or more than three cups coffee and/or six cups tea
   2 one to three cups coffee and/or two to four cups of tea

6 How often do you eat spicy, low-fat foods (like chillies or curries)?

   1 Less than three times a week
   2 More than three times a week

7 Are you: 1 Female or 2 Male

8 And are you: 1 aged under 35 or 2 aged 35 or over

Scores:

0–12: Your metabolic rate may be lower than it could be for helping you get off fat and keep it off. You could benefit by 'revving up the engine' a little.

0–16: Your metabolic rate can probably be increased to help you in your fight against fat.

16+: Your metabolic rate is probably reasonably high for you. There is probably not a lot you can do to increase it—except perhaps more exercise.

4 Weight control or waist control?

Measuring *weight* can be misleading. This is because muscle is twice as heavy as fat. So you might be a short, muscular Mr Universe with low body fat, but come out as obese on standard measures of height and weight. If you exercise to lose fat, as you should, you may find yourself putting on weight in the form of muscle and the water that goes with it, while actually *decreasing* fat, particularly around the middle.

For a man, *waist* is more important than *weight*. And for that reason, you'll notice that we talk about *waist loss*, rather than *weight loss*. We also talk about losing *centimetres*, rather than *kilograms*. In fact, we suggest that you put your scales where they can't be seen and resist the temptation to weigh yourself. To check your progress, use your waist-to-hip measure instead.

Waist circumference: how's your figure?

The best measure of abdominal fat—a 'pot-belly'—used to be the 'waist-to-hip' ratio (WHR) or the size of the waist divided by the size of the hips. A WHR of over 0.9 was regarded as indicating increased risk for disease. However, more recently, it's been found that the measure of waist circumference alone is a good enough approximation of health risk. The cut-off point, regarded as being that beyond which risk increases, is simply 100 centimetres around the waist, irrespective of height. The use of a simple waist measure alone also reduces the complications caused when weight is lost from the whole body. In a small proportion of men, weight loss produces fat loss, not only from the belly, but also from the hips. This is particularly the case with men who have a pear shape. If you lose weight all over, your WHR may actually stay the same, suggesting no improvement in your health profile, and this is not a true representation of what is happening.

These days, then, waist measurement alone is used as our measure of how well you're going. Here's how to do it. Measure around the waist at the navel (see Figure 3). Make sure the tape is parallel to the floor. Relax and *don't* breathe in. If possible, measure at the same time of the day and particularly the same time after eating. Stomach distention after a meal can lead to false readings.

A waist measure of over 100 centimetres in men and over 90 centimetres in women is an indication of increased risk of disease. One hundred centimetres is the long-term goal for all men—irrespective of height. If you're very big—say 150 centimetres around the waist—it may take a couple of years to get down to 100 centimetres, but there's no reason why it can't happen—even if you're 200 centimetres tall! Alterna-

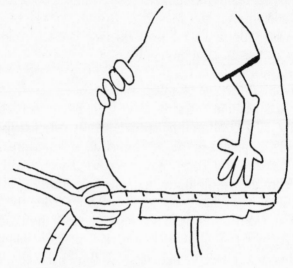

Figure 3:   Waist measurement

tively, if you're very short, the 100 centimetre mark is the general long-term goal. If you're below that, and you still want to shed more fat, you might set your own long-term goal—say, 95 centimetres or even 90 centimetres. Below 90 centimetres it becomes more of an aesthetic issue, rather than a health one.

Most pot-bellied men can decrease their waist size relatively easily with a well-balanced eating and exercise program. You may lose fat from other parts of the body first, such as the neck, chest or buttocks, but there's no need to panic if it doesn't come off the waist first. In most men, though—particularly those with an extended belly—it will usually come off the gut first and fastest. Remember, it's *waist*, not *weight*, you should be interested in.

Big fat lies and how to test them

There are any number of excuses men use to delude themselves into believing they're not fat. But how can you tell without resorting to expensive medical technology? Here are some common excuses and cheap ways to test them.

'I'm not fat—just an OS.'

One way of differentiating muscle from fat is to have a skinfold thickness test. This is painless—a bit like a pinch test with callipers on the arm, leg or stomach. It takes only a couple of minutes and can be carried out by an accredited fitness instructor at any recognised fitness centre. Sports dietitians and a few GPs also use the technique. A small number of doctors and fitness centres may also have other snazzy machines like Bio Impedance Analysis (BIA), which may look better, but they are not always as reliable.

'I'm not overweight—just undertall.'

Weight for height can be tested by using the BMI formula. Take your weight (in kilograms) and divide by height (in metres squared). If your score falls between 20 and 25, you are in the normal range of weight for height. Unless you are short and heavily muscled, over 25 probably means you are fat and over 30 for men and women probably means you are obese.

'It's not fat—it's muscle.'

Muscle is firm, dense and anchored at both ends (to bone), even in the unfit. Fat, on the other hand, is loose, inert and floppy. You can test this with the 'jiggle test'—and a modicum of honesty. Take off your clothes, stand in front of a mirror and jump up and down. If your belly keeps moving after the rest of you has stopped, it's more likely that you're fat.

'It's not a fat stomach—just a sunken chest.'

The 'apple' or android shape is highly associated with the risk of health problems. To measure this, take your waist-to-height ratio. If your score is over 0.5 (for a man), it is definitely not a sunken chest. It's the other.

Why worry about a pot-belly?

There's one good reason. It could take years off your life. But even if it doesn't, it will certainly take life off your years. No fat-bellied man needs to be told that he can no longer move the way he could before he looked like a Christmas stocking half full of melons.

A kilogram of fat needs around 29 kilometres of plumbing (blood vessels) to feed it. And because fat, unlike muscle, is not active tissue, this puts extra strain on the main organ of the body that must supply nutrients to that dead load—the heart.

Imagine pumping air with a foot pump into a flat bicycle tyre. Now imagine doing the same with a flat tractor or truck tyre. The extra work your foot has to do is equivalent to the extra work your heart has to do to pump blood around the body. If the muscles in the foot are weak, they will cramp, seize up and stop you from pumping. In a similar way, if the muscles in the heart are weak, it will seize up too.

A pot-belly can also be a turn-off for women. If you doubt this, ask almost any woman how much she likes an overhanging belly.

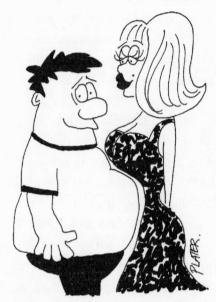

The ideal woman for the slightly-less-than-ideal man.

What causes a pot-belly?

A pot-belly is usually called a 'beer gut'. But beer is unlikely to be a factor in the development of the classic pot-belly. This is because alcohol is used as a primary source of energy in the body. Because it's a toxin, the body needs to get rid of alcohol quickly, and it does this through special metabolic pathways (for technical detail of how this occurs see Appendix 2). When alcohol is combined with fat in the diet, however, the the body is so busy burning up the alcohol that it doesn't burn the fat, which is saved in the fat cells. So the 'beer gut' is probably more accurately defined as a 'beer plus peanuts' or a 'beer plus chips' gut—or just a 'fat' gut.

For this reason, the GutBuster program not only suggests, but *insists*, that you don't go off alcohol as part of the program. This is because the program has to be based around things you can do (and enjoy) for life. Most men who give up alcohol will take it up again at some stage. And when they do, everything else will be dropped. As we've seen, alcohol itself is not fattening. If you learn to live with it, by reducing fat intake in ways discussed in Chapter 7, you can lose waist at the rate of 1 per cent a week while still drinking up to four standard-sized drinks a day. That should be enough to make you want to read on!

Smokers have been found to have more of a 'pot' than non-smokers, even when alcohol and exercise are taken into account. It's not yet known why this is so, because smokers are often lighter than non-smokers or ex-smokers. But even smokers who do not weigh much may have a hazardous layer of fat around the waistline.

The many ways of measuring body fat

The use of weight scales as a measure of body fat is limited because weight includes water, muscle, bone and organs as well as fat. There are now a number of techniques available to measure fat more specifically. Some are expensive and complex; others are as simple and cheap as a tape measure. Ranging from high to low in accuracy, these include:

- *Underwater weighing* measures the displacement of water, and bases calculations on the principal that fat floats, to measure total body fat.
- *Radioisotopic techniques* use total body water or lean body mass as estimated from total body potassium. They require injection of radioactive material into the body.
- *Multiscan Computed Tomography* (CT scanning) and *Magnetic Resonance Imagery* (MRI) are complex and expensive technologies able to detect visceral (internal) as well as subcutaneous (or surface) fat.
- *Bio Impedence Analysis* (BIA) is based on the ability of tissue of different density to be penetrated by an electric current. Fat content is then worked out using a computer model.
- *Near Infra-Red Analysis* uses a low-frequency light beam on the skin. The type of tissue from which this is reflected will determine a colour of the light spectrum and fat content can be calculated from this.
- *Skinfold callipers* measure subcutaneous fat at various sites and use a derived formula to convert these to a percentage of total body fat. The skinfold measurements are accurate but the formula is not.

> • *Waist-to-Hip Ratio* (WHR) is a measure of abdominal fat taken by dividing waist measurement by hip measurement. Ratios over 0.9 in males and over 0.8 in females are in the high risk range.
> • *Body Mass Index* (BMI) is a formula using weight divided by height squared (kg/m^2) where the normal range is 20–25.

Researchers have found that a man who gives up smoking, and doesn't compensate by exercising more or changing his food pattern, can expect to gain an average of about 2.3 kilograms of weight. His 'pot' will increase slightly, but only about one-fifth of what would be predicted from the increase in total body weight.

On the other hand, those who start or restart smoking have been found to lose an average of about a kilogram in weight. However, their pot-bellies still tend to increase. This contrasts with non-smokers, whose pot-bellies decrease with any weight loss.

There's also a relationship between the size of a pot-belly and the number of cigarettes smoked. The more cigarettes a man (or a woman) smokes daily, the greater the size of the belly compared with the hips. So the claims of those who say that smoking helps keep their weight down are negated by the fact that they store extra fat right where it is most dangerous.

A big eater can have a 'big belly' and be fat all over. A smoker, on the other hand, can have a 'tobacco belly' and be thin everywhere else. He looks like a straw with a pea stuck in it!

Individual differences

Unless you came down in the last shower, you've probably also noticed that some people lose fat more easily than others. Men, we have said, can usually lose it quicker than women.

Even between men, however, there are differences. For example, our work shows that men who lose fat most easily are those who:

- store it mostly around the gut (the pot-belly)
- are more 'apple-shaped'
- have put most of their extra fat on after their teen years
- have parents who are not excessively fat
- are not obese, or excessively fat.

Those who have most trouble losing it:

- have fat families
- were overfat before their teens
- are more 'pear' shaped or 'box' shaped (i.e. fat all over).

From research carried out with working men in Australia, four different classifications have been identified in relation to body fat and how easily different men can lose body fat. The four types are listed in the box below.

Male fat types

When it comes to weight control, working men can be divided into four groups, according to research carried out in Newcastle, Australia. These are:

---

1   Weight 'cyclers': so called because, although they
    have put on fat since their youth, they seem to be
    able to shed it regularly, and with relative ease.
    When they decide to lose weight, 'cyclers' do it by
    going on a diet (mostly an unbalanced one), by
    cutting back or eliminating alcohol or, much less
    commonly, by a planned increase in exercise.
    Cyclers approach weight loss with a free and easy
    attitude and frustrate their spouses no end because
    of the ease with which they can do it when they
    want to. 'Cyclers' generally have pot-bellies. The
    majority of overweight men fit this category.

2   'Perennials' are perpetually trying to lose fat and
    are able to do so (with much effort and denial) to
    a certain point at which weight plateaus and goes
    no lower. More effort, no matter how serious,
    seems to produce little result. Understandably,
    'perennials' experience anxiety and frustration and,
    at the extremes, even pent-up anger at 'the world'
    in general and the 'Jack Sprats' (see below) in
    particular.

3   'Deniers' accept that they are overweight but, at
    least outwardly, don't care about it. There are two
    sub-categories in this group:
    (a) 'Pseudo-deniers' are those who use defensive
        forms of denial such as humour, abuse,
        argument, bravado, etc. to hide what seems
        to be a genuine anxiety about being
        overweight.
    (b) 'Real deniers' are those who seem genuinely
        not to care. They represent only a small
        proportion of overweight men.

4 'Jack Sprats' are a rare breed who seem to be unable to get fat. These are the whippets of the workforce who are spoken about in almost mythological terms because of the huge amounts they have been known to eat and drink without ever putting on weight. Although 'Jack Sprats' make up only a tiny proportion of middle-aged and older men, every man appears to know or have known one.

If you fall into the first category of being a *weight cycler*, you need the GutBuster program. Losing weight and then regaining it, losing it again, regaining it once more, and so on, is worse for health than staying fat. However, if you can lose weight easily using the wrong methods, you'll have no difficulty losing weight once and for all using a well-balanced program.

If you fall into the second category of a *perennial*, you'll also benefit from the GutBuster program, although perhaps not as much as someone from the first category. You might also need some other professional help from a dietitian or your doctor, to make allowances for your individual differences. Such differences are also important in selecting the *eating* and *exercising* programs that best suit you. You'll notice this as you go through the GutBuster program.

If you fit the third category and *deny* you have a weight problem, we hope that reading this book will help you accept that a pot-belly deserves some attention.

If you're a 'Jack Sprat', you're probably either very active or you may be genetically programmed with a high level of fidget activity. Small movements such as shifting from one side of your bottom to the other while sitting, moving legs, arms, shoulders, head and hands a lot and generally getting out of a chair fast and walking with a large expenditure of energy all add up to fidget activity. Researchers in the United States have found that we burn up anything from 100 to 900 Calories a day in this type of activity. A 900 Calorie-a-day fidgeter tends to distress his mates with his obvious jumpiness, but lower levels of inbuilt fidget activity may go unnoticed. However, they mean you have a constant fat-burning mechanism working for you. This fidget activity is already apparent in young infants and is almost certainly inherited. If you picked the right parents, you may thus be able to eat much more than other people because your small movements carried out for around sixteen hours a day burn up more calories.

Some apparent 'Jack Sprats' may eat a lot when they're with their mates, but then automatically cut back on what they eat for the next couple of meals. Their overall intake is thus less than what it sometimes appears to be.

Ways not *to lose weight*

It's often thought that men don't care about being overweight the way women do. Although some studies have shown this to be the case, our research shows differently.

Men *are* worried about having a 'gut'. They don't like being asked by their kids if they're 'pregnant' and when they're going to produce a little brother or sister.

And they don't enjoy being less able to do the things they could when they were leaner.

Yet when most men try to trim down, they go about it the wrong way. Some typical mistakes they make are shown below.

Mistakes men make

- *Skipping breakfast or lunch*: Breakfast stimulates metabolism so you burn up more calories for the whole day. All meals need energy to be digested. Skipping meals means you burn calories at a slower rate.
- *Giving up alcohol*: If you give up something enjoyable, you're likely to take it up again at some point. When you do, everything else is likely to go by the wayside. Alcohol itself is not fattening, so learn to live with it and enjoy it, if that's your desire.
- *Drinking soft drinks or fruit juices*: Most men think beer is fattening. They don't realise that sugary soft drinks and even pure fruit juices have as many calories as beer.
- *Cutting out carbohydrates*: Potatoes and bread are good, low-fat, complex carbohydrate foods. Cutting out carbos will just make you tired and depressed and make exercise more difficult.
- *Eating too much fat*: Fats are far more fattening than anything else you can eat. They are also more 'addictive' than other foods. Cutting back on fats can decrease the appetite.
- *Fasting or crash dieting*: This may cause short-term weight (water) loss, but lowers metabolism and increases body fat in the long term.

- *Being inactive*: Activity burns fat not only while you are doing it, but afterwards as well.
- *Concentrating on weight, instead of fat*: It's waist fat that most men should be concerned about. Weight can be misleading.
- *Doing sit-ups for a fat stomach*: These work muscle, not fat. They'll leave you with a tight fat stomach instead of a loose fat one!

Smoking and fat loss

If you've never been a smoker, you can skip this section. But if you are a smoker, or a recent ex-smoker, there are some important points you need to know if you want to lose fat from your gut.

Smokers can and do put on weight when they quit. There are three possible reasons why this occurs:

1 Smokers who quit are less nervous and fidget less. This means they use up fewer calories—and it all adds up.
2 Smokers who quit eat more. The increase in calorie intake after quitting might be due to:
   (a) more sensitive taste-buds. Smoking decreases some taste sensations and quitters often find food tastes so good that they eat more.
   (b) 'nerves'. Smoking gives you something to do with your hands and this may be replaced by eating, usually sweet and fatty snacks.
   (c) greater appetite. Smoking depresses the appetite so quitters usually feel extra hungry.

(d) the fact that a cigarette often signifies the end of a meal. Quitters sometimes don't know when to stop eating.

Ex-smokers generally benefit most from a controlled diet plan with small, frequent, healthy meals—at least over the first few months—to make sure they don't gain weight. Controlling appetite after giving up smoking is another matter.

3 Nicotine speeds up the body's resting metabolic rate (RMR). Smokers therefore burn up more energy. This is often increased further by drinking lots of coffee, and while it may have a small positive effect on weight control, it can also induce stress. Nicotine and caffeine have a combined effect. Even after quitting, smokers' caffeine levels remain higher than those of non-smokers, causing nervousness, edginess and the desire for another cigarette for its calming effect.

Most research shows that if quitting smokers want to avoid gaining weight, a combination of a low-fat diet and a moderate increase in exercise is the best way of doing it. Exercise can also act as a substitute for smoking and may decrease the desire for nicotine. Learning new habits may also help (see Part II of this book). If the problem is severe, short-term drug treatment can be effective and safe, but you'll need to see your doctor for this.

Recommendations for quitters who want to lose fat

- Be aware of when and where you eat and try to avoid any increases in food intake.
- If necessary, use a good safe, reliable government diet plan devised by qualified people.
- Increase the small amounts of physical activity you do—such as walking more, not using a remote control for the TV, beating eggs by hand, using stairs instead of lifts, etc. It all adds up to burn up more calories.
- Slow down or cut back on caffeine intake (mainly coffee, but also be careful with tea and cola) at least over the first three to four weeks.
- Snack on fruit, vegetables or bread, or even small quantities of sweet foods without fat (like jelly beans or meringue without cream), rather than sweet or fatty foods.

Part II

The four-step approach to losing a pot-belly

5 Step 1: Changing habits

Life is short, so there's hardly enough time for it all to be spent thinking about every physical action we make. Habits stop us from having to do that. We develop habits so we don't need to think about every action. Habits are ways of responding that become automatic and enable us to do, and think about, other things while we're doing them.

There are two main types of habit: one seems most characteristic of men and the other is more common in women. The first type, behavioural habits, are simply learned actions. They develop when a response is conditioned to a stimulus. These are simply bad ways of acting. The second type of habit is a cognitive habit, which is a learned way of thinking. If it develops from a cycle of negative thinking, it can become simply a bad way of thinking.

From a health viewpoint, habits can be good or bad. Basic hygiene habits, such as cleaning your teeth or washing your hands, are good behavioural habits. But much of what we do in relation to food and exercise can become bad habits and cause increases in body weight. For example, we often eat not because of hunger, but because of the cues that we have learned to associate with eating.

One of the best examples of this occurs when an advertisement comes on midway through a television program. For some people, this offers the opportunity to get up, stretch their legs, obey a call of nature, actually talk to their partner or kids and generally do things that they were too glued to the screen to do during the program.

If you were to get up on a couple of occasions and, without thinking, grab some food, or a beer or coke from the fridge, you'll soon associate ad breaks with eating or drinking. Most of us think of eating or drinking as a form of reward and, as psychologists know, reward for a response very quickly conditions that response to the stimulus for it. In other words, in this case:

ad break = going to fridge = food or drink = reward

Therefore, in future, through the process of conditioning:

ad break = food

It's a bit like a rat in a Skinner box. A Skinner box is basically a rat cage where the rat learns that, when a light comes on, it will get food if it presses a bar. Psychologists call this 'operant conditioning', and it's a way of forming an automatic habit very quickly. Pretty soon, it's the light, not pressing the bar, that becomes associated with eating, just as it's the advertisement on

TV, not *hunger*, that makes you want food. So every time there's an ad on TV, you learn to eat—whether you're hungry or not!

Most people don't eat when they're hungry.
They eat from force of habit.

The ad break, of course, is only one example. There is a range of other habits we pair together every day that contribute to getting fat—for example, always having a biscuit with a cup of tea, eating chips or peanuts with a beer, jumping in the car whenever we need to go anywhere or buying a chocolate bar when we pay for petrol. They are all unconscious little habits that add calories in the energy equation.

The second type of habit, more characteristic of women—at least in relation to weight control—is cognitive habits. These can lead to a vicious cycle of eating. dieting, starving, then binging, as shown in Figure 4. This pattern is usually not common in men, but if it's a problem for you, you'll need to break the cycle to have any positive effect. Give yourself permission to eat, but mostly eat those things that we recommend here.

Modifying habits

There are two main points to the formation of habits that need to be tackled if you really want to break the habit cycle.

1   *Recognising and understanding habits*: To do any-
    thing about them, you need to be aware of the

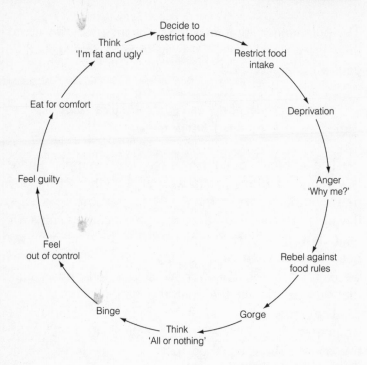

Figure 4: The vicious cycle of obesity

situations and stimuli that make you do those things
in automatic gear that you pay for in manual gear
later. To become aware of habits you have to 'stalk'
them, as a hunter stalks his prey. By watching these
actions, from the outside, you can learn to stalk out
the little things you do during the day that are
working against you losing fat. Some hints for doing
this are shown as a check list on page 64.

2   *Breaking the habit cycle*: Once you've stalked your
habits and appreciated what they are and how they

occur, the next stage is to break the stimulus–response cycle. Again, psychologists know that to break this cycle you either remove or replace the reward. In this case, the reward is invariably food (or sometimes slothfulness). If the habit is eating at TV ad breaks, the solution is to *do something* other than eating at these times. Because this might be too sudden a change, you may need an intermediary stage such as having a glass of water at ad breaks instead of eating. If your usual response is a cup of tea with two biscuits, the intermediate stage may be cutting back to one biscuit or changing to a piece of fruit before moving to the second stage which is to have tea without biscuits.

As many habits are unconscious, it's important that once these are stalked, the consciousness level remains high. One way of doing this is to record every time

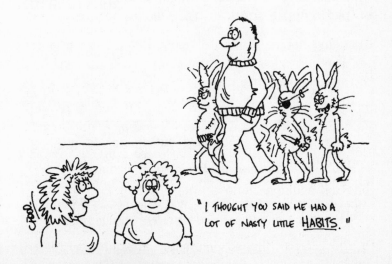

" I THOUGHT YOU SAID HE HAD A LOT OF NASTY LITTLE <u>HABITS</u>. "

that you do or don't respond to that particular habit within a day, and then check these recordings to see if the habit decreases over time. If you trust yourself to remember, there may be no need to record. Instead, remind yourself every time the stimulus occurs to make sure the response doesn't.

Some of the most common habits in men that work against a flat stomach are:

- eating snacks while drinking beer
- drinking beer or soft drinks *with fatty meals*
- raiding the fridge in the middle of the night
- getting the kids to do things for you if they involve any effort
- always eating several courses when you're eating out
- thinking that meals eaten out are different—perhaps more of a treat—than those eaten at home
- associating soft drink with thirst
- picking up a snack on the way home from work.

Changing habits is often difficult. But it's not impossible. It requires learning some simple skills that will help you unlearn inappropriate habits. Try yourself on some of the tips in the table below.

Tips for changing eating habits

1. **Change the eating/drinking environment**
I do this

Eat only in designated places and when sitting down ☐
Set regular eating times and don't eat outside these ☐
Plan snacks and meals ahead of time ☐

Dissociate eating from other activities
(e.g. watching TV, reading) ☐
Don't have fatty foods in the house ☐
Record your food intake ☐
NEVER shop when hungry and ALWAYS
stick to a shopping list ☐
Avoid places where you think you have to eat or
drink ☐

2 **Change the manner of eating or drinking**
Chew slowly and put utensils down between
mouthfuls ☐
Pause in the middle of a meal for a few minutes ☐
Savour foods: enjoy each bite ☐
NEVER eat until 'stuffed'—just until satisfied ☐
Allow at least 20 minutes for eating a meal ☐
Don't get in a round of drink buying ☐
Clean plates directly into the garbage and remove
immediately ☐
Just have a main course—skip the entree,
appetisers and sweets ☐
Come to terms with, and enjoy, not feeling stuffed
full of food ☐

3 **Change food choices**
Cut snacks in half ☐
Serve only amounts planned ☐
Pre-plan portion amounts when entertaining ☐
Drink *low-alcohol* beer/*low-calorie* soft drinks ☐
Share sweets if you have to have them ☐
Increase the variety of foods you eat ☐
Have low-fat snacks planned and 'ready to go' ☐
Use herbs/spices instead of high-calorie dressings
and condiments ☐

Use low-calorie ingredient substitutes (e.g. low-fat milk) ☐

4 Change activity patterns

Walk, wherever possible—don't drive or ride ☐
Change TV channels manually ☐
Do it yourself—don't ask the kids to do it ☐
Walk up stairs—don't use the escalator or lift ☐
Join a gym or walking club if that's your scene ☐
Take up an active sport or recreation ☐
Do active tasks or errands around the house ☐
Get a partner to walk with you ☐
Walk a set distance especially for fat loss—every day ☐

Your score:

0–18: There is a lot to do. Add those 'no' scores to your life in future.

19–28: Your habits are reasonable, but you can do better.

28–36: Your eating habits are not your problem. Read on.

The hunger scale

Hunger is the biological urge to eat. Appetite is a socially conditioned response to food. To make sure you're eating when you're hungry, rather than just when you think you should, get used to rating your feelings of hunger on the following scale.

8   Beyond full—totally stuffed
7   Very full
6   Slightly full
5   Feeling satisfied

4 No hunger
3 Slightly hungry
2 Hungry
1 Ravenous

Never let yourself get too hungry—that is, 2 or less—because this means you'll have no resistance to eating all the wrong things. But also try not to eat if your rating is 4 or above, because this means you're satisfying appetite, not hunger.

6 Step 2: Moving more

Most fat control programs emphasise diet. But more people are beginning to recognise the importance of movement, or exercise. Physical activity burns up fat, rather than promoting muscle loss as occurs with many diets. Also:

- Movement can be enjoyable (who ever enjoyed a diet?).
- Movement can be used to 'trade off' food and drink intake (you don't see too many fat marathon runners).
- Going 'on a diet' implies that sometime you've got to come off it. Activity is something that can be made part of your life.

Exercise—or movement?

The first point to make about exercising for waist loss is that it is not necessarily the same as exercising for fitness. In fact, exercise is the wrong term. That's why we've called this chapter 'Moving more'.

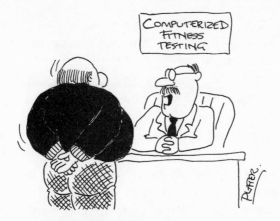

" IT RECOMMENDS THAT YOU KEEP YOUR INSURANCE PAID UP. "

Movement of any kind uses up energy. And we know that energy, if not replaced from food, is taken from the body in the form of fat. Energy is measured in calories (or kilojoules, if you prefer—1 Calorie = 4.2 kilojoules).

But it's wrong to think that it's only the energy that is used up during movement that helps the weight loss process. You may read in popular magazines that walking a kilometre burns 60–70 Calories and that this is the equivalent of only a single slice of bread. But it's the other things that go with activity that are most important. Research has shown, for example, that exercise may increase the metabolic rate by 10–20 per cent over 24 hours. So while walking an extra kilometre a day may burn off around 70 calories, the 24-hour effect of that could *theoretically* be a 10 per cent increase in the metabolic rate, or more than twice the direct effect over a day.

Also, while a planned exercise or fitness program will obviously burn fat, you don't have to go to the level of joining a gym or taking up aerobics, or even pounding the pavement in a pair of joggers. It could simply mean walking a little more instead of going everywhere in the car, getting a little more active with the kids or mowing the lawn instead of paying someone else to do it.

It's the little bouts of energy use that add up and become important, in the same way that, as we described earlier, 'fidget' activity can burn so much energy. Not surprisingly, it's also been shown that the overweight tend to take the easy way out when physical effort is required. Videos of overweight kids playing tennis show that they try to 'grow a longer arm' to hit a ball that's out of reach rather than move their feet to get to the ball.

Similarly, many people become overweight because they own every labour-saving device that comes on to the market—portable telephone, remote control video, electric can-openers and many other gadgets. But what do you do with the time you've saved? Most people spend their spare time sitting watching television and do very little that's active—apart from lifting food and drinks to their mouths. So they get fat.

For the working man, the problem is built into the system. Even a decade or two ago, manual workers were much more active. They walked, lifted, carried or dug, all manually. Now there are few workplaces that aren't mechanised, so that most actions are done by machine without any need for the worker to move—apart from pulling levers or pressing buttons. There are very few 'working men' left if 'work' is defined as an activity involving energy use.

Technology and development are also against us. Professor Phillip James from the Rowett Institute in Scotland has estimated that the average person in the mid-1990s was using approximately 800 Calories a day less than in 1980. This is the equivalent of reducing walking by around 10 kilometres a day, and it comes mainly from having machines do everything for us. It's clear from this that, although the mind may desire it, the human body is not yet ready for the technological revolution.

So how do we overcome this? The sad fact of modern life is that what nature gives on the swings, it takes when the roundabout stops. The human body was made to move. When it doesn't move, it gets fat. If you want to get rid of that fat—without going back to the days when there were few little luxuries of life—you need to make a planned effort. You have to do it yourself. Modern life won't do it for you.

As we have said before, this doesn't mean you have to train like an athlete to be fit. Strange as it may seem, walking a kilometre burns roughly the same amount of energy as jogging a kilometre. Admittedly it takes a little longer, but if you don't have to compete, why run when you can walk?

You don't have to 'bust a gut' to lose a gut.

Vigorous activity can also be quite dangerous for someone carrying too much fat. If your heart is weak (and a deconditioned heart often is) and you make it pump blood vigorously through all the extra 'plumbing' you've developed to service large mounds of fat, the load can be potentially fatal.

So let's forget bust-a-gut exercise and think about moving more, in big ways and little ways, and all the time throughout the day.

Movement—are you doing enough?

Over 30 per cent of people in the United Kingdom, the United States, Australia and New Zealand are currently totally sedentary—they participate in no physical activity other than the bare minimum required for survival. Test your own activity level by truthfully answering the following question.

Do you currently participate in any regular acivity or program, either on your own or in a formal class, designed to improve or maintain your physical fitness or body weight?

If your honest answer is 'no', there's a fair chance that your excess fat is due to your lack of movement. There's certainly room for improvement. If your answer is 'yes', there may still be room for improvement, particularly if you like your food and would like to continue having a drink (see Chapter 8 on trading off).

There are two main types of movement we're interested in. The first is an increase in incidental movement carried out during the normal day. The second is a planned program of increased physical activity.

Incidental movement means moving your body during the day when you might otherwise take the easy way out. Walk up the stairs instead of taking a lift; walk to the shops instead of driving; mow the lawn instead of paying someone else to do it—even put the remote control on top of the TV and change the channels by hand. Increasing incidental movement requires a change in mindset. You should start thinking of all forms of movement as an opportunity, not an inconvenience. Hence, instead of parking the car as close as possible to the food pick-up in your shopping centre and cursing the guy who gets in closer than you, park at the back of the carpark and take the opportunity to burn off some extra fat.

Start thinking of movement as an opportunity
not an inconvenience.

Although it may not sound like much, the energy used up in incidental movement adds up. It can also help to increase your metabolic rate, or the rate at which your body burns energy at rest. This means it could take much less time for you to lose those extra centimetres.

Here are some other simple rules for incidental exercise:

- Don't ride when you can walk.
- Don't sit when you can stand.
- Don't ask others to fetch things when you can get them yourself.
- Don't use a lift or escalator when you can use the stairs.
- Don't use power tools when you can use manpower.

- Get off public transport before your stop and walk the rest of the way.
- Park your car some distance from your destination and walk.

Incidental movement should form the base of your physical activity pyramid (see Figure 5). If you're very big, have an injury or just simply find it difficult to walk or do any other form of exercise, this may be all you need until such time as you lose some weight, repair your injury or have more time. Provided it's combined with the proper eating program referred to in Chapter 8, and provided the incidental movement you do is more than you're doing now, you *have* to lose weight. Don't under-estimate the power of incidental movement!

Planned movement involves selecting an 'aerobic' activity of your choice and carrying it out at least every other day. Aerobic activities are those which use the large muscles of the body over an extended period. They include such activities as walking, jogging, swimming, cycling, rowing, aerobics, circuit training, callisthenics, etc.

Walking is probably the most under-rated, but the easiest, cheapest and most enjoyable aerobic exercise for most people. The formula is simple:

To 'lose a gut', walk (anywhere, anytime, with anyone) for 3–4 kilometres every day. It doesn't matter whether you go late at night or early in the morning; on a treadmill or on the road; with a mate or with your dog—just walk! Recent research shows that it also doesn't matter whether you do it all at once, or whether you do four lots of 1 kilometre walks throughout the day. And the speed is not important. The main thing is the distance. Of course, as you get fitter, by simply walking, you'll be able to go faster (and probably want to go faster). If this is the case, fine. But in the first instance, just cover the distance.

Most men have the mistaken belief that, unless they exercise to the point of exhaustion, it's not worth it. But that's not correct. A re-evaluation of data from exercise science research in the 1980s has shown that weight loss is related to the duration and frequency, and not necessarily the intensity, of exercise.

If you have injuries, or you're too heavy for weight-bearing exercise such as walking (that is, where you're carrying your own body weight), try swimming, get on an exercise cycle, or walk on a mini-trampoline (available from any sports store) in your lounge room. You can even watch TV while you do it. But remember, this type of weight-supportive activity is never as good as the weight-bearing type. Swimming, for example, is not a good fat-loss exercise because the body weight is supported and it's therefore less energetic (unless, of course, you can't swim!). Still, it's better than nothing, so if that's all you can do, or all you like doing, do it—and try to cover about one quarter of the distance of walking, that is, around 1 kilometre a day. Walking or wading through water is a good exercise, which also takes the pressure off damaged hips or knees, so if you live near a beach or shallow pool, you could try this.

Here are some other tips for planned movement:

• Select only an aerobic exercise, or exercises, you enjoy.

- If it's walking (perhaps the best exercise) walk 3–4 kilometres a day (or four lots of 1 kilometre).
- If it's some other exercise, try to do it (or them) for at least 30 minutes (or three lots of ten minutes) each day.
- Exercise *before* a main meal (with the exception of swimming, it reduces the appetite).
- Vary your exercise (either different ones each day or a different route each day).
- Exercise with a partner—to keep each other motivated.
- Record how much you do each day—in distance or time.
- Plan ahead, and make sure you don't miss out.
- If it suits you, go for a walk before eating in the morning. You may burn more fat that way because your sugar stores have gone down overnight and the body calls more on fat for energy.

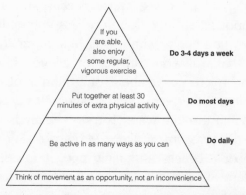

For greatest weight loss, aim to go as high as you can on the pyramid

Figure 5: The physical activity pyramid
Source: Australian Government, National Physical Activity Guidelines 1998

The values of various exercises (with ratings out of 10) for waist control for men are shown in the table below:

Rating of the value of exercises (out of 10) for waist loss in men[*]	
Walking	10
Jogging	10[***]
Aerobics	10
Cycling	8
Circuit training (gym)	8
Skipping/stepping	8[***]
Squash (average level)	8[***]
Surfing (body or board)	7
Tennis (singles)	6
Rowing/canoeing	6
Golf	6[**]
Mini-trampolining	5
Swimming	5
Dancing (ballroom)	5
Gardening	2

[*] Ratings are based on levels of convenience, injury potential, and enjoyment (for a set time each day) as well as effectiveness. Higher scores are best.

[**] Golf as a form of walking would be rated higher if it was carried out daily.

[***] These exercises are not recommended for the very obese.

For a planned program of extra movement to be successful, it has to be enjoyable—something you feel comfortable doing for life. So it's important that you make the right selection from the start. If you haven't exercised for years, it's often hard to know what you like.

There are two ways to cope with this. You could

try a range of different activities—perhaps walk one day, swim the next, try a mini-trampoline the next. That way you'll soon find out what you do and don't like doing. Or do the questionnaire in Appendix 3 called the 'Exerselector'. Follow the instructions and fill out the scores to find out just which exercise(s) you may be best suited to, even though you may not have known it.

It's vital that you choose an exercise that you can be happy doing for the rest of your life. If you don't, and you only choose something for a short period to get weight off, your gut is bound to return.

Different types of exercise have advantages and disadvantages, so they may suit some people and not others. You can get an idea of this from the table below.

Advantages and disadvantages of different types of exercise for fat loss

Exercise	Advantages	Disadvantages
Walking	Comfortable; convenient; non-weight supportive and therefore high energy use	Not good for knee, ankle, foot injuries; may be difficult in some areas
Jogging	Takes less time; can be 'addictive', good to do with mates	Can be uncomfortable; dangerous for overweight; can cause injury; too much like work

Exercise	Advantages	Disadvantages
Swimming	Comfortable; few injuries; good for very overweight because weight is supported; good in summer	Doesn't burn as much energy (because weight is supported); not as good for women (because their high fat level makes them more buoyant); can be taken too easily; cold in winter; sometimes inconvenient
Cycling	Enjoyable; comfortable (because weight is supported) for the very overweight; can be done at different intensities	Not as good for fat burning as non-weight supportive; can hurt knee, hip problems
Tennis/Golf	Enjoyable; social; not too energetic; Lots of walking (particularly if you're not very good)	Golf may be difficult to play 18 holes every day (unless you're lucky)
Aerobics	Enjoyable; social; high rate of energy use; muscle tone as well as fat loss	Requires some coordination; needs good instructor; can be too hard
Skipping	Convenient; high rate of energy use	Boring; can cause leg injury; needs coordination; difficult to carry out for long enough
Squash	High rate of energy use; enjoyable	Dangerous for the overweight; can cause back injury; too vigorous—recommended only for those who are fit and not overweight; not recommended for fat loss

Exercise	*Advantages*	*Disadvantages*
Rowing	Good for those with lower body injury; can be portable (rowing machine)	Can be boring

Getting feedback: the FATT principle

We've said that moving to lose fat doesn't have to be the same as exercising to get fit—you don't have to get fit to lose fat. So training for fitness may be different from moving for fatness. Of course, once you start to lose some weight from any type of movement, you might start to get fit, and then you might want more. But at first, the main thing is moving for fatness, rather than exercising for fitness. The two different outcomes are explained by the acronyms in the table below.

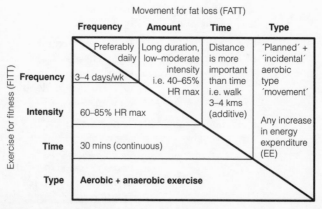

Figure 6:   The FITT/FATT table

For getting rid of fat, the acronym spells out the following:

- **Frequency:** You should be walking (or doing some other form of planned exercise) on six, or preferably even seven, days a week.
- **Amount:** We've set the distance required at 3–4 kilometres a day. But remember, this doesn't all have to be done in one session each day.
- **Time:** Speed is not important. The main thing is the distance covered, not the speed. However, when you get fitter, you might be able to cover the distance at a faster speed and therefore have more time for doing other things. It's up to you.
- **Type:** Walking is the best and most convenient fat-loss exercise. Failing that, other activities such as jogging, skiing, aerobics, skating or circuit training will do. These are all aerobic, which is important, because it's only during aerobic activity that fat is metabolised. Anaerobic exercise (such as sprinting, lifting weights or very vigorous short activities should be reserved for sports training, not for fat loss, because they burn more sugar than fat.

If weight-bearing activity is a problem, weight-supportive activities can be used for planned movement. These include cycling, swimming, rowing, surfing, mini-trampolining, or other types of movement you might dream up. To anticipate your next question, sex is not an effective fat-loss activity unless you're an extremely talented bedroom athlete, as it requires 30–40 minutes of elevated heart rate using the large muscles of the body—and don't kid yourself!

Some of the principles used for fitness training can also be useful to the waist watcher, particularly as the fat starts to peel off. These were also shown in Figure 6. The acronym that's often used for fitness training is FITT. (frequency, intensity, time and type), so if it's fitness as well as fat loss you're after, check yourself against the menu outlined below:

- **Frequency:** Your planned activity program should preferably be carried out every day if you really want to lose fat, but at minimum, every second day. Make sure you don't miss two days in a row.

- **Intensity:** The appropriate intensity of the effort can be gauged from your heart rate. This can be measured at the radial pulse at the wrist (at the base of the thumb). Count the heartbeats for 30 seconds and then multiply by two to get a pulse rate per minute. The average resting pulse for a man should be around 72 beats per minute and for a woman 80 beats per minute. Resting pulse can be used as a form of feedback, because as you get fitter and lose some fat, this is likely to decrease.

  The pulse rate for carrying out an organised exercise program should be around 120–130 beats per minute for safety and effectiveness. As you get older, however, this will decrease, so for a 60-year-old, a pulse rate of 100–110 for fat loss is adequate. Another formula is to work out 50–60 per cent of the maximum heart rate (MHR), where

$$MHR = 220 - age$$

  This gives a value for improving aerobic conditioning and doesn't necessarily apply to weight loss. As we've said, movement is the key factor for fat loss, not intensity.

- **Time:** The daily amount of time for exercise should be around 30 minutes a day. However, if 30 minutes in one hit is not possible, several bursts of ten minutes will do. For greater benefits, spend more time doing gentle aerobic exercise. However, the longer you exercise, the greater the risk of injury, so we suggest that, at least in the early stages, you take it easy and be content with 30 minutes until some weight is lost.

- **Type:** The type of exercise necessary for fat loss is aerobic. This involves using the large muscles of the body over an extended period at a faster heart rate than occurs with walking, swimming, jogging, cycling, etc. The larger the muscle group involved, the greater the effort and hence the greater the potential waist loss. For fitness, though, you'll also benefit from some anaerobic activity—that is, some short bursts of vigorous activity mixed with your aerobic exercise. Because this puts extra pressure on the heart, fitness type activity is different from that needed for fat loss.

Enjoyment

To be of any permanent value, an activity routine has to be something you can do for life. So if you don't like what you're doing, try something else. Of course, you should first give it a fair go. For anyone who's overweight and unfit, any form of exercise can be a bit unpleasant at first. But once you get used to it, it should start to lose any air of punishment.

Test yourself on the scale below to make sure you're doing the right thing.

Physical activity enjoyment scale

Rate how you feel at the moment about the physical activity you've been doing:

1	2	3	4	5	6	7
I hate it						I enjoy it

1	2	3	4	5	6	7
I feel bored						I feel interested

1	2	3	4	5	6	7
I am not at all absorbed in it						I am very absorbed in it

1	2	3	4	5	6	7
I find it tiring						I find it energising

1	2	3	4	5	6	7
It's very unpleasant						It's very pleasant

1	2	3	4	5	6	7
I feel bad physically while doing it						I feel good physically while doing it

1	2	3	4	5	6	7
I'm very frustrated by it						I'm not at all frustrated by it

1	2	3	4	5	6	7
It's not at all stimulating						It's very stimulating

1	2	3	4	5	6	7

It doesn't give me
any sense of
accomplishment

It gives me a
strong sense of
accomplishment

1	2	3	4	5	6	7

I feel as though I would
rather be doing something else

I feel quite happy
while I am doing it

Scores:

<30: You're definitely doing the wrong exercise routine (for you). Look for a change in routine before you lose interest completely.

30–50: Although you're moderately suited to your routine, you could possibly find some other forms of exercise that would give you more satisfaction.

50+: Your exercise routine is suited to you. Keep evaluating it to make sure it stays that way.

Exercise and body shape

Different exercises have different effects on body shape. Basically, there are three main types:

1 those that result in a *loss* of body mass (i.e. 'shrinking' exercises)
2 those that result in a *gain* in body mass (i.e. 'bulking' exercises)
3 those that result in a decrease of fat, but an increase in muscle (i.e. 'toning' exercises).

The different types of exercise and their effects on body mass are shown below.

Exercise effects on body shape

Body mass loss Shrinking exercises	Toning exercises	Body mass gain Bulking exercises
Walking	Aerobics	Weight training
Jogging	Circuit training	Sprinting
Distance cycling	Swimming	Shot-put
Cross-country skiing	Rowing	Hammer-throw
Soccer	Gymnastics	Sprint rowing
Tennis (singles)	Wrestling	
Badminton	Canoeing	
Hockey	Surfing	
Volleyball	Callisthenics	
Dancing	Windsurfing	

As can be seen from the arrows, combining exercises from different categories will have an effect, depending on which category is carried out most. For example, combining walking with aerobics will cause fat loss and improve muscle tone. The more walking, the greater the fat loss; the more aerobics, the greater the muscle tone. Combining a toning and a bulking exercise will cause an increase in body mass and is therefore of little value for the man wanting to lose fat. Fat loss is obviously greatest using a shrinking exercise. However, once fat starts to be lost, a toning exercise can help tighten up those parts of the body that used to wobble. For anyone who has a pot-belly, bulking exercises are likely to be of little benefit.

Exercise in the cold

It's a popular myth that if you sweat a lot while you exercise, you'll lose more fat. This leads a lot of men to jog or walk in a tracksuit, heavy clothing or body wrap, or to try to exercise more in hot weather or during the hotter parts of the day. It might surprise you to know that this is exactly the wrong way to go. While any exercise burns energy, research in Canada has shown that exercise in the cold is particularly efficient for using fat as an energy source (in contrast to carbohydrate), and hence burns up more fat than similar exercise in a warm climate. The fat-burning effect of the cold is even more obvious in obese people.

It's thought that cold weather has this effect by stimulating catecholamines (a type of hormone) which are involved in stress, but also have a lypolytic, or fat-burning, effect. The combination of cold and exercise then generates an effective level of catecholamines without excess physical stress on a person who is relatively unfit.

Again, this doesn't imply that you have to exercise in a refrigerator to get the most benefit. It does mean, though, that those times when you may feel least like exercising, such as early mornings in winter, may indeed be the best in terms of greater fat loss. Certainly, any idea of doing yourself a favour by wearing thermal underwear or a heavy tracksuit while going for a walk in the middle of a hot summer's day should be dismissed. Also, if you're planning on a weight-loss holiday to Hawaii (irrespective of what you eat) you might be kidding yourself—instead try Sweden,

Switzerland or Antarctica. Indeed, the whole idea of 'fat farms' being located in the warmest parts of the country is off the beam. Weight-loss clinics of the future are more likely to be situated in the snowfields.

7 Step 3: Eating differently

It's a popular myth that losing weight means eating less. It is more likely to mean eating differently. But if this is done correctly, you can actually end up eating more food and still losing fat. Specifically, this means decreasing the amount of fat you eat and increasing foods high in both fibre and carbohydrate. You'll notice we haven't said 'diet', because we'd like you to wipe the word from your vocabulary. It's a nasty four-letter word and can actually help to make you fatter over the long term. Start to think more in terms of a lifetime eating plan, or LEP, rather than a DIET. In particular, look at the following:

Decreasing fat in the diet

One gram of fat provides your body with 9 Calories, whereas a gram of carbohydrate or protein has only 4 Calories. Alcohol provides around 7 Calories per gram, but as we've seen, this is burned up early in the energy cycle. Fat is the most fattening of the nutrients.

Hence it's fat in food which is the big danger. When we eat fat, it takes very little effort for the body to convert that fat into body fat. By contrast, when we eat carbohydrates, it takes much more effort for the body to convert them to fat. In fact, under normal circumstances, the process of conversion of carbohydrate to fat, called *de novo lipogenesis*, does not play a big part in humans as was once thought—particularly in males. Instead, the body uses carbohydrates to increase metabolic rate or warm the body (great if you've decided not to overdress).

Some scientists also think that fat might be addictive, and that the craving some people have for apparently sugary foods could really be a craving for fat. The 'sweet tooth' may be a misnomer. It may be a 'fat tooth' rather than a 'sweet tooth'. When you think about it, all the foods people commonly ask for to satisfy their sweet tooth—cakes, biscuits, pastries, desserts, chocolates, ice-cream—are high-fat foods.

Fat people often crave high-fat foods. One researcher manipulated the fat and sugar content of foods and asked people to rate which ones they preferred. He found that fat people only liked sweet foods when they also contained fat. Thin people were the opposite. He concluded that fat people love fatty foods, while thin people don't.

Fat in food is higher in calories than other nutrients, can give you a craving and is more likely to be stored as fat on the waist.

Chemically, some of the appeal of foods is due to the smell of hot fat and the creamy sensation high-fat foods produce in the mouth. High-fat foods also seem to have a satiating effect after eating that is qualitatively different from other foods. A fatty steak or chop, for example, leaves a different feeling of fullness than a carbohydrate food such as a steamed potato. In fact, recent research on a satiety index has shown that fats don't fill you up at the time of eating (although you may feel full later) so you tend to eat more. Have you noticed that you can always fit in some chocolate at the end of a big meal, but not a dozen oranges or apples, which may have the same number of calories?

It's reasonable, as some scientists have proposed, that fats may create a craving for more of the same—in other words, they make you hungry—thus increasing the appetite for food in general, and fatty foods in particular.

The other side of the same theory is that going off fatty foods should decrease the appetite for them and thus the amount of calories you consume. Certainly the experiences of people who cut back on fatty foods suggest that one of their main effects comes from a reduced desire for fat. This may not happen straight away, but may take several weeks to develop. Most people who don't eat fatty foods regularly also find them sickening. For example, those who never eat the fat on meat find it revolting. Those who give up eating it soon feel the same way.

Some fats contain essential fatty acids and are important. But too much fat can also be a health hazard. Eating too much saturated fat increases the levels of blood cholesterol and triglycerides, can raise blood pressure and may promote diabetes. Too much of almost any kind of fat, including polyunsaturated fats, may also be a cause of gallstones and certain types of cancer. The safest fat is probably olive oil—a product that has been used for thousands of years. But even olive oil has the same high calorie level as any fat. It makes sense to buy expensive, strong-flavoured olive oil. The cost will help reduce consumption and just a few drops will add flavour to foods such as salads. The oils in fish are also healthy, and are unlikely to be fattening. And that means all seafoods—including prawns, lobsters, crabs and oysters—provided they're not fried, crumbed or battered. For that reason, a principle of the GutBuster program is that you can eat anything that comes from the sea.

Identifying fat foods

It can be difficult to identify foods that are high in fat. Although some fats are visible, many of the fats in modern foods are hidden and you wouldn't guess how much fat they contain. For example, some fast-food burgers have over 60 per cent more fat than a traditional Australian burger, but they don't seem fatty. And who would have guessed that a meal of quiche and salad can have six times as much fat as a piece of lean steak and some vegetables?

Another common misconception is that vegetable oils are less fatty than animal fats. Almost everyone assumes vegetable fats are healthier than animal fats. Some are, but vegetable oils may come from a source such as palm kernels or coconuts which have more saturated fat than beef dripping or lard. Other vegetable oils are partially hydrogenated during processing and

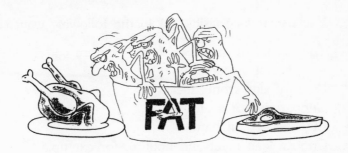

this converts some of their original unsaturated fats into saturated ones. Even worse, processing can produce fats known as *trans fats*, which are even worse for health than saturated fats. Labelling products as containing no cholesterol is also confusing, as many of these foods are high in fat.

Sources of fats in the Australian diet

Source	% contribution to fat intake
Oils, margarines, cooking oils	43
Meat	22#
Dairy products	19*
Poultry	5
Grains	3
Nuts	4
Eggs	1
Seafood	1

\#   Now available in lean cuts (e.g. new pork, trim lamb, lean beef)
*   Most are now available in low fat. Cheeses are still a problem. Ordinary cheeses are around 33 per cent fat; reduced fat cheeses 25 per cent; but some of the new cheeses such as Bega Super Light or Devon Seven have around 7 per cent fat and still taste like cheese. Beware of cheeses which state 'low cholesterol', as many are still high in fat.

You can reduce visible fat in the following ways:

- Trim all fat off meat, preferably before you cook it so it is not so tempting.
- Remove skin from chicken.
- Choose fish or seafood.
- Buy reduced-fat ham.
- Choose lean meat and poultry, for example:
  - fillet, topside, lean mince (the most expensive)
  - turkey or chicken breast
  - veal or new-fashioned pork
  - trim lamb cuts
- Cook with less fat by
  - grilling
  - microwaving
  - dry-frying
  - barbecuing
  - steaming
- Choose low-fat (cottage or ricotta) or reduced-fat cheeses.
- Use spreads thinly—or preferably skip them altogether.
- Use minimal oil in cooking (no more than one tablespoon for four serves, preferably olive oil).

Dietary fat questionnaire	
1 How often do you eat fried food with a batter or breadcrumb coating?	
six or more times a week	4
three to five times a week	3
one to two times a week	2
less than once a week	1
never	0

2 How often do you eat gravy, cream sauces or cheese sauces?

six or more times a week	4
three to five times a week	3
one to two times a week	2
less than once a week	1
never	0

3 How often do you add butter, margarine, oil or sour cream to vegetables, cooked rice or spaghetti?

six or more times a week	4
three to five times a week	3
one to two times a week	2
less than once a week	1
never	0

4 How often do you eat vegetables that are fried or roasted with fat or oil?

six or more times a week	4
three to five times a week	3
one to two times a week	2
less than once a week	1
never	0

5 How is your meat usually cooked?

Fried	4
Stewed or goulash	3
Grilled or roasted with added oil or fat	2
Grilled or roasted without added oil or fat	1
Eat meat occasionally or never	0

6 How many times a week do you eat sausages, devon, salami, meat pies, hamburgers or bacon?

six or more times a week	4

three to five times a week   3
one to two times a week   2
less than once a week   1
never   0

7 How do you spread butter/margarine on your
   bread?
   thickly   3
   medium   2
   thinly   1
   don't use butter or margarine   0

8 How many times a week do you eat chips or French
   fries?
   six or more times a week   4
   three to five times a week   3
   once or twice a week   2
   less than once a week   1
   never   0

9 How often do you eat pastries, cakes, sweet biscuits
   or croissants?
   six or more times a week   4
   three to five times a week   3
   once or twice a week   2
   less than once a week   1
   never   0

10 How many times a week do you eat chocolate,
   chocolate biscuits or sweet snack bars?
   six or more times a week   4
   three to five times a week   3
   once or twice a week   2
   less than once a week   1
   never   0

11 How many times a week do you eat potato crisps, corn chips or nuts?

six or more times a week	4
three to five times a week	3
once or twice a week	2
less than once a week	1
never	0

12 How often do you eat cream?

six or more times a week	4
three to five times a week	3
once or twice a week	2
less than once a week	1
never	0

13 How often do you eat more than a small serve of ice-cream?

six or more times a week	4
three to five times a week	3
once or twice a week	2
less than once a week	1
never	0

14 How many times a week do you eat more than a small piece of cheddar or other hard cheese, semi-soft cheese such as camembert or cream cheese?

six or more times a week	4
three to five times a week	3
once or twice a week	2
less than once a week	1
never	0

15 What type of milk do you drink or use on breakfast cereal or in cooking?

condensed or evaporated	4

full-cream	3
full-cream and reduced fat	2
reduced-fat	1
skim	0

16 How much of the skin on your chicken do you eat?

most or all of the skin	2
some of the skin	1
none of the skin/I am a vegetarian	0

17 How much of the fat on your meat do you eat?

most or all of the fat	2
some of the fat	1
none of the fat/I am a vegetarian	0

Scores:

0–17: Your fat intake is relatively low. Keep it that way.

18–39: Your fat intake is moderately high. Reduce it if you want to lose weight.

40+: Your fat intake is high. This will have to be reduced if you want to lose weight, feel better and improve your health.

- Buy low-fat dairy products—skim or lite milk and low-fat yoghurt.
- Avoid fatty meats such as salami, devon or sausages (unless they are special low-fat types).
- Keep fatty foods such as chocolate, crisps, cakes pastries, etc. for a weekly treat or special occasions.
- Use no-oil and low-fat mayonnaise or try a little lemon juice or vinegar instead.
- Roast meat on a rack so the fat can drip away.
- Keep invisible fats to a minimum. These include:

- the fat in cakes, biscuits or pastries (including croissants)
- the fat in chocolate, nuts or crisps
- the fat in pies and sausage rolls
- the fat in toasted muesli
- the fat in fast foods.

Recognising rip-offs

We are not going to give you a long lecture on the nutritional value of what you eat. But you need to know a few facts about food and drinks so you can enjoy yourself without doing too much damage. There are also many crazy ideas about foods and you may be restricting yourself unnecessarily on some foods and not enough on others. Let's see how well you score on the big fat rip-off. Try the following quiz.

The fat questionnaire		
	True	**False**
1 Potatoes and bread are more fattening than meat.	T	F
2 Butter is more fattening than margarine.	T	F
3 Jogging a kilometre burns more calories than walking.	T	F
4 Raw sugar and honey are less fattening than white sugar.	T	F
5 Switching from beer to spirits will help you lose weight.	T	F
6 Light beer is less fattening than standard beer.	T	F
7 Polyunsaturated fat is less fattening than saturated fat.	T	F

8	Olive oil is less fattening than other oils.	T	F
9	Walking is better than sit-ups for losing a pot-belly.	T	F
10	A glass of beer is more fattening than a glass of cola soft drink.	T	F

Answers:

1 F. It's what you put on the bread and potatoes that is fattening.
2 F. They have the same calories.
3 F. Walking just takes longer!
4 F. There's no difference in calories in these 'natural' sweeteners.
5 F. Unless you drink less—and don't add mixers.
6 T. Alcohol level also indicates calorie level.
7 F. They're both the same—gram for gram.
8 F. It is better for your cholesterol, but all oils are equally fattening.
9 T. 'Aerobic' exercise burns fat. Sit-ups tighten muscle.
10 F. Most (not diet) soft drinks are just as high or higher in calories than beer.

Increasing fibre

Dietary fibre comes in plant foods. Unlike most parts of our food, humans cannot digest dietary fibre in the small intestine. Dietary fibre therefore passes to the large intestine where most of it is digested by 'good' bacteria, producing some valuable chemical effects in the process.

The different types of dietary fibre are usually described as insoluble or soluble. Both types of fibre tend to create a full feeling so you feel satisfied. High-fibre foods are rarely fattening, mainly because they are so bulky that it is difficult to eat too much of them.

Some hints for adding fibre to your diet are:

- Use wholemeal or wholegrain bread.
- Choose wholegrain cereals such as wholemeal pasta, brown rice, wholegrain crispbread, rolled oats, and wheat, barley or oat breakfast cereals.
- Add wheat bran, oat bran, rice bran, barley bran or mixed bran or wheatgerm to cereals, or to casseroles or soups.
- Eat the skins of fruits and vegetables where appropriate—for example, have potatoes in their jackets, and eat the skin on apples.
- Eat more vegetables and fruit.
- Try wholemeal varieties of crumpets, muffins, scones, raisin bread and hot-cross buns.
- Eat more dried peas, beans and lentils (e.g. soy beans, kidney beans, baked beans, Lima beans, etc.).
- Drink plenty of water with your high-fibre diet.
- Eat fibre with protein (e.g. a chicken and salad sandwich—not just chicken).

Eating for fat loss

The ideal way for anyone to lose fat is to think of foods in three categories:

1 foods you can eat in large portions
2 foods which are fine in moderate portions
3 foods which are best in small portions.

Don't assume you know which foods fit into each category because there are a lot of myths about foods suitable for anyone wanting to lose weight. For example, most diets are designed so the weight loss is due mainly to water and muscle tissue. You can achieve this sort of weight loss fast if you avoid high-carbohydrate foods such as bread, cereals and potatoes. This is the basis of most popular fast weight-loss diets but it does *not* mean that bread, cereals and potatoes are fattening. It means that if you don't eat these foods, you'll temporarily weigh less because you'll lose water from the body. If you keep up the absurdity of skipping bread, cereals and potatoes, you'll also lose some lean muscle tissue. The scales may give you some pleasure, but your lighter-weight body will probably still have all its fat. After a few weeks, or whenever you go back to eating some of the carbohydrate your body needs for energy, the lost water will return and you'll regain most of the lost weight. The lost muscle won't reappear unless you spend time exercising to rebuild it.

As a measure of fat loss, weight scales are useless, at least in the short term. Throw them out.

Ignore all fast weight-loss diets. They don't work, at least not for more than a couple of weeks. Afterwards, you're fatter than ever. If you examine most of them, they are some kind of variation on a low carbohydrate diet. They may make seductive statements such as 'eat whole chickens and still lose weight' or 'eat all the pasta you like', but closer inspection reveals a different story. It turns out that when you eat chicken, that's all you can eat. Lots of pasta sounds good, but the fine print says you can't have anything with the pasta. In practice, few people will eat much straight dry pasta without sauce, cheese or butter.

No matter how tempting the latest miracle diet may sound, it won't work. Millions of fat people are hoping for a miraculous diet which will dissolve their excess fat with little effort and lots of fatty food. There's no miracle and no real alternative to sensible eating. However, a balanced program doesn't mean you have to go hungry. Read on.

Foods you can eat in large portions
This includes all vegetables (raw or cooked), fruits (but not juices because they've lost their dietary fibre), breads and cereals (with at least some as wholemeal or wholegrain products because they have more fibre and are therefore more filling) and seafoods.

No one ever grew fat on vegetables—and that includes potatoes. To gain 1 kilogram of fat from eating potatoes, you'd need to eat 95 potatoes each weighing 130 grams! However, if you deep-fry your potatoes as chips, or bake them in fat or oil, or smother them with butter, margarine or cream, the added fat *will* add to your waistline.

It would be difficult to eat enough fruit to make you fat. You can safely eat three to five pieces a day without worry. We restrict fruit juices because they've lost their fibre and it's easy to drink your way through piles of fruit which has been juiced to yield all its calories. It might not make you fat, but it could stop you losing

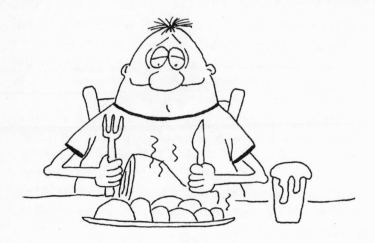

fat. Always eat fruit with its fibre. Another GutBuster principle is '*Never drink anything you can eat whole*' (of course, with the exception of cow's milk!).

Contrary to popular belief, you won't get fat from eating bread. It's not the bread, it's the spread that causes problems. Breads of all kinds—including English-style muffins, bread rolls, pita bread, flat breads, raisin bread or even crumpets—are all low in fat. As mentioned earlier, the idea that bread is fattening developed from crash diets where the aim is to achieve a lower reading on the scales rather than actually losing fat. By the same token, you shouldn't eat whole loaves of bread in one sitting, or your body will never get round to burning its fat for energy.

With rice and pasta, you can also let your head go—as long as you don't coat them with lots of fat. Steamed rice is fine. So is straight pasta. But some pasta dishes, such as lasagne or fettuccine with a creamy sauce have heaps of fat. Unless you use a special low-fat recipe, it's best to stick with sauces made from tomatoes, mushrooms, capsicums, any other vegetables, herbs, some wine (if you like) plus seafoods or lean meat or chicken.

Breakfast cereals (which can be eaten at any time of the day) are also not likely to make you fat—unless you choose some toasted mueslis which have a lot of added fat, or you add full-cream milk to them. Choose cereals with ingredients that don't include coconut oil, vegetable oil, palm kernel oil or any other type of fat. And use a low-fat milk. It also makes sense to choose cereals that are mostly cereal, rather than the highly sweetened cereals that can have more sugar than cereal. Sugar is a carbohydrate, but it doesn't have the nutritional benefits of cereals. High-sugar cereals are also low in fibre, so they're not so filling.

Seafoods are great indulgence foods and, as we've seen, you can eat large portions without problems. Grill them, barbecue them, cook them in the microwave, on a wok or in a Chinese bamboo steamer—but don't dip seafoods in batter and deep-fry them. You can also use canned fish, but choose those in brine or spring water rather than the varieties soaking in oil.

Fish and all seafoods are low in fat. If you've previously been warned off prawns because of their high cholesterol content, relax. Less than 30 per cent of the cholesterol in prawns is absorbed by the body and they have almost no saturated fat. When some lucky volunteers were fed prawns, lobster, crab, octopus and various other seafoods and their cholesterol levels were measured, the old assumptions that some seafoods increased cholesterol were proved wrong. Foods which increase cholesterol are those high in saturated fat.

Foods to eat in moderate amounts
Growing children and teenagers can handle plenty of lean meats, chicken or turkey, eggs and dairy products. For adults, moderate quantities of these foods are still important to provide protein, iron, zinc, calcium and many vitamins, but you don't need a lot—and any excesses will easily be converted to body fat. A small lean steak is fine; a huge T-bone that hangs over the edge of the plate may produce a similar overhang over your belt. There's no need to become vegetarian, but remember that growing kids need plenty of protein— grown men need less.

Always buy meat which is lean. Fat on meat will easily become fat on you. It also makes sense to remove the fat from meat *before* cooking it. Crisp golden fat is harder to resist so cut it off while it's a cold, white, unattractive lump of fat, rather than after it's cooked.

Chicken is also best without its skin. You can buy skinless chicken breasts, thighs and legs—all meat and no waste. If you find it impossible to do without chicken skin, strip off half the skin and throw it away before sitting down to enjoy the rest. Turkey is a lean product and it's not so difficult to throw away its skin. Turkey ham and turkey salami are also available in some delicatessens and supermarkets. Both are lean products that are useful on sandwiches or in cooking to add flavour, and turkey salami has only one-tenth the fat content of many meat salamis. Turkey breast is suitable for anyone trying to eat less fat and wanting a touch of luxury. Emu is also lean.

Many dairy products come in low-fat versions. If you've never liked low-fat milk, start mixing up three-quarters regular milk and one-quarter low-fat milk. Each week, increase the proportion of low-fat and, before you know it, you'll be using 100 per cent low-fat milk. Low-fat yoghurt is a good snack food, although not always popular with men. Almost 50 per cent of men in some countries have never even tasted yoghurt! Give it a try—it makes a great dessert with some fruit, and a good dollop of yoghurt on top of an oven-baked or microwaved potato is excellent.

Foods to eat in small amounts
The worst foods for fat loss are fats. Sugary foods are not much better because it's so easy to eat or drink such large quantities before feeling full. Foods packed with sugar *and* fat, such as chocolates, pastries, pies, cakes, biscuits and many desserts, are a disaster for anyone wanting to lose fat. This doesn't mean you can never have any of these foods, but it does mean you should keep them for special occasions, or at least have only a small serve. Fried foods are also a nightmare, often loaded with more fats than you'd get in dozens of slices of bread.

Eating habits

Go for filling not fattening
Most foods that are filling are not fattening. Strangely enough, many people get it the wrong way round and

deliberately avoid good, filling foods. A bowl of porridge, for example, has no more calories than a bowl of some flimsy cereal. But the porridge is so filling that it sticks to your ribs and reduces your desire to fill up on biscuits at morning tea time.

Foods with plenty of fibre are often filling. Take potatoes, for example. They're an excellent source of fibre without being fattening—unless you have them loaded with fat as chips, or smothered in butter or margarine. Fruit, wholemeal bread, baked beans, pasta, rice and cereals are all filling, high-fibre foods that you can and should include in your diet.

Sugar, on the other hand, doesn't fill you up at all. You won't feel any fuller after drinking a can of soft drink with ten to twelve teaspoons of sugar than you will after drinking the same volume of diet soft drink or water. And if you choose water, soda water or mineral water, you'll also avoid the acidity of diet soft drinks which is a hazard for tooth enamel.

Many fast foods aren't very filling either. They're designed to be that way, with very little filling fibre and plenty of slippery fat so they'll slide down your throat easily without making you feel full. Most people think fast food means you don't have to stand in a queue very long to buy it. Fast foods are really foods that are fast to eat. Their high-fat and low-fibre content means they need little chewing. When you eat fast, you tend to eat more. It's good for business, but it's not so good for the size of your belly!

Eating sensibly doesn't mean starving yourself. It means choosing high-fibre, high-carbohydrate, low-fat foods so you can eat more. Take a look at the comparisons in the box below:

Calorie comparisons in foods		
1 T-bone steak with fat	=	15 slices of bread
200 g bar of chocolate	=	11 slices of bread + 1 banana + 1 apple + 1 orange + 1 punnet of strawberries
1 Mars bar	=	4 slices of bread
1 Danish pastry (100 g)	=	4.5 slices of bread
1 iced fruit mince slice	=	4 slices of bread + 1 apple + 1 pear
1 Big Mac	=	3 big thick salad sandwiches
1 bucket of hot chips	=	5 medium potatoes
2 meat pies	=	2 cups baked beans on 2 slices of toast + 1 banana + 2 oranges + 1 large apple

To help sort out common confusions about food, meals and nutrition, we've put together a few food facts.

Breakfast—why you should eat it
Overnight, your body is metabolising energy slowly. When you get up, your metabolism increases slightly and you start burning some more calories. When you eat breakfast, however, your metabolism really speeds up.

It's easy to busy yourself getting ready for the day and skip breakfast. Missing breakfast means you go like a slug all day. We don't see fat people who overeat at breakfast. Many fat people eat very little breakfast and they don't start their bodies metabolising energy fast. Most fat people could do with more breakfast—and a little less dinner.

Breakfast is probably the most important meal of the day for the overweight. Don't miss it.

Lunch—don't miss it

Breakfast won't last you until dinner. Lunch is an important meal too. It doesn't need to be large, or cooked, but you shouldn't skip it. People who skip lunch tend to snack about 5 or 6 pm, often on chocolates or chips—foods which easily increase body fat. It would be better to have a few sandwiches or a bread roll or a pita bread filled with chicken and salad topped off with some fresh fruit at lunchtime. A liquid lunch tempts many men, but it won't give you the energy to keep going at top pace all afternoon. It's a good rule to make sure you never drink alcohol without having something to eat. Alcohol is also likely to put you to sleep for the afternoon.

What about dinner?

The evening meal is the best chance most of us get to relax and take time over a meal. That's fine. Taking time to eat is good for your digestion. It's also good for your GutBuster program to have the right balance of foods on your dinner plate. Some people think anyone wanting to lose fat will get only a saucerful of food. Nothing could be further from the truth. It's not *how much* you eat, but *what* you eat. If your plate is two-thirds meat and one-third vegetables, change the balance to two-thirds vegetables and one-third meat. It makes much better nutritional sense: your plate will still be full and the vegetables are filling. In fact, you can eat lots of vegetables—any kind (except fat-soaked chips). Cook vegetables in the microwave to preserve their nutrients or steam or stir-fry in a non-stick pan.

Most men aren't too fussed about skipping dessert. If you're different and you love your sweets, look at our suggestions at the end of this chapter.

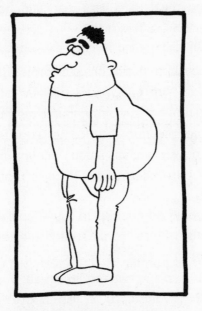

THE CONSEQUENCES OF NOT
READING THE SMALL PRINT OF
THE "GUT REDUCING DIET."

Eating out

Meals at restaurants and clubs or from fast food establishments are often very fatty. If you can, avoid fried foods, especially foods which have been dipped in batter and fried. Ask for your fish or prawns to be grilled or barbecued. Ask for salads to be served with their dressing separate so you can add just a little for flavour rather than having a salad drowned in fatty dressing. You might also have to ask for vegetables to be served without margarine or butter.

There are some fine lean meats around these days and most restaurants serve them along with chicken or turkey. Game meats are very lean and healthy and it would make good sense if we could get back to eating game animals.

Take-away tucker

Unfortunately, much fast food tends to be high in fat and low in fibre. However, there are some more healthy choices that can be made.

Best choices at the take-away bar	Worst choices
Plain hamburger	Hamburger with the lot
BBQ or char-grilled chicken (remove skin)	Fried or crumbed chicken
Pizza with bread crust (try vegetarian)	Pan pizza with extra toppings
Bread rolls/sandwiches	French fries/chips
Kebabs	Kebabs with extra meat
Grilled fish and salad	Fried fish and chips
Toasted sandwiches	Pies/sausage rolls

At the club

Roast dinners	Lots of meat/few vegies
BBQ steak (sandwich size) and salad	Fried steak and thin chips
Grilled seafood/oysters natural	Fried seafood platter
Casseroles with lots of vegetables	Casseroles with pastry and chips
Sandwiches/rolls	Pies/sausages/bacon
Ask for extra vegetables/salad	Avoid side order of chips

Chinese/Asian

Short/long soup	Fried dim sims/spring rolls
Chow mien/chop suey	Sweet and sour dishes
Stir-fried dishes	Chicken in lemon sauce
Steamed fish	Crumbed/battered seafood
Steamed rice/noodles	Fried rice/noodles
Steamed rice	Fried rice
Order a dish of steamed vegies	Peking duck

What about cholesterol?

Cholesterol is a waxy type of fat that is essential in small quantities for the body's hormones, nerve and brain cells. Cholesterol also helps us digest fats and use certain vitamins. Problems arise when the body makes too much cholesterol and the excess is deposited in the arteries, making it harder for the heart to pump blood through.

Some people's bodies make more cholesterol than others. Once again, it helps if you picked the right parents! However, no one makes cholesterol out of air, so you can't lay all the blame on your parents. We make cholesterol in the body when we eat too much saturated fat. The actual cholesterol in foods such as eggs or prawns is much less of a problem.

A lot of confusion over cholesterol comes from food labels proudly boasting 'no cholesterol', even though the food may have as much as 80–100 per cent fat or may never have had any cholesterol anyway. In some countries, there are guidelines for manufacturers which state that 'no cholesterol' claims should not be made on high-fat foods. Unfortunately, the guidelines are ignored by some food manufacturers. If you have high cholesterol (ask your doctor to check your level), try to cut back on all saturated and trans fats. When you can't avoid fat, use a small quantity of olive oil.

Thankfully, alcohol doesn't increase cholesterol, although it can increase another hazardous type of fat in the blood called triglycerides. Being too fat will increase the risk of high cholesterol and high triglyceride levels.

Losing fat around the gut helps reduce high levels of cholesterol. And, as we've seen, the best way to lose waist fat is to eat less fat. So this program can kill two birds with one stone.

Vitamins—do you need them?
Foods such as fruits, vegetables, legumes, high-fibre breads, grains and cereals, low-fat dairy products, seafoods and lean meats have plenty of vitamins and very few people need to take supplements. In fact, if your diet is low in vitamins, it makes sense to fix the diet rather than continue eating junk foods and adding a pill.

Many men take a fizzy vitamin B tablet after a night on the town, hoping the vitamins will stop the hangover. They won't. Alcoholics are often deficient in vitamin B1 and giving them this vitamin helps prevent irreversible brain damage in them. However, this doesn't mean that everyone who has a drink should take extra vitamin B. By eating more bread, especially wholemeal, and by following the guidelines in this book, you should not need extra vitamins. There's no real evidence that vitamins can prevent a hangover.

Some people believe that soils don't give plants the nutrients they need to make vitamins. This is not true, and official analyses of foods show high levels of vitamins. Even fast foods contain vitamins, although the same analyses show high levels of fat in fast foods, and this is a much greater problem.

Suggestions for meals and snacks

Breakfasts
Choose any of the suggestions listed below, adding tea or coffee if desired. We haven't specified how much toast or any other food you should eat. This is *not* a diet and there's no weighing or measuring. Have reasonable serves, according to how active you are, how genuinely hungry you are and how much waist you have to lose. But don't skimp on breakfast or you'll reduce your metabolic rate and more than make up for your frugality later. Better to eat at breakfast time. Here are some breakfast suggestions:

*   wholewheat or other wholegrain breakfast cereal with fresh fruit and low-fat milk
*   toast, preferably wholemeal, with tomato or low-fat spread and vegemite

- boiled, poached or scrambled egg with grilled tomatoes
- toast, preferably wholemeal
- grilled tomatoes, mushrooms and canned sweet corn (hot)
- toast, preferably wholemeal
- baked beans on toast
- fruit
- grilled fish with lemon
- wholemeal toast
- large bowl of fresh fruit salad with low-fat yoghurt
- toasted wholemeal English-style muffin with low-fat spread and a little honey
- potatoes, cooked, sliced and browned on a non-stick pan with sliced onions, grilled tomatoes
- toast, preferably wholemeal.

Lunches

Most people have their main meal in the evening. If it's possible to have your main meal at lunchtime, do so—you'll have more time to burn off its calories before the day ends. If you take your lunch to work, you have plenty of choice in what you take. If you buy your lunch, try to avoid fast foods such as pies, pasties, sausage rolls, chips and battered foods. If you dine in a restaurant, there are usually some good choices to make. Here are some examples of each:

Taking lunch from home
- sandwiches or rolls or pita bread plus fresh fruit. Skip the spread, if possible. Suitable sandwich fillings include salad plus any one of:

- chicken
- turkey (with cranberry sauce, if desired)
- turkey ham
- turkey salami
- lean roast beef (add some mustard or horseradish)
- lean pork (with apple sauce, if desired)
- veal (with chutney, if desired)
- lean ham (with mustard or pickles, if desired)
- a slice of cheese (preferably fat-reduced)
- cottage cheese
- hard-boiled egg
- tuna
- salmon
- a large salad and bread roll (preferably multigrain or wholemeal) plus fresh fruit
- soup (either taken in a thermos or heated at work) and bread roll (preferably multigrain or wholemeal) plus fresh fruit or fruit salad
- piece of cold chicken, potato salad (use low-fat yoghurt instead of mayonnaise in dressing), bread or roll and fresh fruit.

Eating lunch at home
Any of the ideas above, or:

- baked beans on toast plus a piece of fruit
- grilled tomato and cheese on toast plus fruit
- home-made soup (e.g. pea, vegetable, potato, barley and vegetable, tomato or pumpkin) with toast and fruit
- stuffed potatoes and salad (bake or microwave whole potatoes until soft, scoop out centres, mash

with some mustard or chilli or chopped mushrooms
and herbs, pile back into potatoes and reheat).

Buying take-aways for lunch
*   sandwiches, pita bread or rolls with fillings as listed
    earlier, plus fruit. Ask for your sandwiches to be
    made without butter—you won't notice the differ-
    ence on a freshly made sandwich
*   Lebanese bread with felafel, salad or tabbouli
*   a quarter of a barbecued chicken (try to remove
    skin) plus a bread roll and some fresh fruit salad
*   kebab plus bread and salad
*   hamburger, preferably from a small store, plus fruit
    salad
*   fish, grilled rather than fried, plus salad and fruit or
    fruit salad
*   toasted sandwiches (ask for no butter) plus fruit
*   Asian take-away—suitable choices would be any-
    thing steamed; any seafood dishes (not in batter or
    fried); stir-fried beef, chicken, pork or seafood;
    chow mein; long or short soups; curries (without
    coconut milk) with steamed rice
*   tacos with beans and salad (ask for no cheese or
    sour cream) with fruit salad
*   vegeburger with fruit.

Lunch in a restaurant or club
*   small steak (e.g. fillet or small rump) with vegetables
    or salad and bread roll (skip the butter and ask for
    no chips)
*   oysters, barbecued prawns, grilled or barbecued fish
    or any seafood which is not fried or in batter. If
    you have the choice of chilli and garlic with your

barbecued seafood, take it. Remember chillies might help a little

- chicken or turkey breast with vegetables or salad plus bread roll (skip the butter)
- pasta with sauce of tomatoes, mushrooms, capsicum or any other vegetables or seafood (include any spicy ingredients such as chilli or herbs but avoid creamy sauces and lots of cheese) with salad
- curries and rice (avoid too many curries based on coconut cream).

Dinners

Dinner is usually the most relaxed meal. Some men stuff themselves with too much dinner, sit (or snooze) in front of the television for the evening and wonder why they get fat! We don't need a heavy meal at the end of the day. But that doesn't mean you have to look at a tiny plate of food. Your plate can still be heaped—but with more vegetables, and not too many fatty foods. The basic principles of dinner should be:

- Eat lots of vegetables, any kind, but don't add butter or margarine. Make sure the vegetables take up three times as much space as the meat.
- Potatoes are no problem except for chips.
- Rice, pasta or other cereal or grain foods are fine.
- Meat must be lean—all fat removed before cooking.
- Try to eat fish or other seafoods (canned or fresh) often.
- Take the skin off chicken or start with chicken breast or thigh fillets or skinless legs.

Cooking

Some cooking methods are better for your waistline
than others. The less fat you use, the better—so barbecuing, grilling, steaming, using the microwave or
cooking in a non-stick pan are better than frying in fat
or oil.

Barbecuing is a great way to cook, but it also makes
sense to switch to cooking some lower-fat foods. Fish,
prawns, octopus, chicken kebabs, lean beef and trim
lamb are all great on the barbecue. You can also thread
some tiny tomatoes, mushrooms, pieces of zucchini,
onion or capsicum on skewers and add them to the
barbecue. With some bread and salad, you can enjoy
a great barbecue without a heap of fat. (If using wooden
skewers, soak them in water for 15–30 minutes before
using so they won't burn.)

Whenever you can avoid adding fats or oils, do so.
Sometimes, however, you need a little oil—for example,
if you're browning onions. Here's a tip for using less
oil. Start with a good-quality, heavy-based non-stick
frying pan. Once heated, pour in about a teaspoonful
of oil, then add onions or anything else you need to
brown. Cover with a loose-fitting lid. By making a
heavy pan hot, you can brown an onion in a quarter
of the oil it takes if you pour the oil into a cold pan.
Olive oil is the healthiest oil to use, but remember that
every oil—including those labelled 'light' or 'no cholesterol'—is 100 per cent fat.

Stir-frying is a good cooking method when you're
in a hurry. There are two ways to cut down on fat.
One is to heat the wok or pan before you start adding
any oil or food (as mentioned above). The other is to

stir-fry using chicken stock instead of oil. Get your wok or pan good and hot, add a little chicken stock (about half a cup) and then toss in whatever you're going to stir-fry (chicken or pork or fish or beef and vegetables). Toss or stir the mixture while it cooks. The chicken stock makes it glossy and adds plenty of flavour. Add a little soy sauce for flavour (preferably the salt-reduced one).

Microwave ovens are great because they make cooking quick and easy. You can cook many dishes in a microwave faster than you can dash out to buy take-aways. Vegetables are also good cooked in the microwave. Don't add any water and you won't lose any flavour—and you'll also keep most of the vitamins. Simply place vegetables in a microwave-safe dish, cover and cook according to your microwave directions. Don't forget how easy it is to cook potatoes in the microwave too. A hot potato makes a great snack when you're feeling peckish. The microwave is also good for rice, pasta, fish or to cook extra vegetables which you can then reheat later if you're feeling hungry.

Sauces can be included in low-fat foods. Use various vegetables, fruits, herbs, wine, different vinegars or mustards as flavourings with stock.

Dessert
The best dessert is fruit—fresh, stewed or canned (choose brands without added sugar). If you want something more, try one of the following:

- baked apples (core apple, fill centre with raisins, prunes or chopped dried apricots, make a small slit

around the skin in the middle of the apple to stop
it splitting and bake in a moderate oven for 30
minutes or microwave on high for 3–5 minutes or
until soft)

- fruit crumble (for 4 serves, use 2 cups pie pack
canned fruit, sprinkle with cinnamon and top with
a mixture made by combining $1\frac{1}{2}$ cups rolled oats,
with $\frac{1}{4}$ cup each of wheatgerm, brown sugar and
processed bran cereal and two tablespoons of
reduced-fat butter; bake in a moderate oven for 30
minutes)

- fresh fruit salad mixed with low-fat yoghurt (if using
a flavoured yoghurt, select one without sugar) and
a little cinnamon or chopped ginger. Stand for at
least 30 minutes to allow flavours to blend

- low-fat ice-cream with rockmelon and passionfruit,
or with fresh berries

Snacks

Some people don't need to eat snacks. Others, especially those who have physically demanding jobs, get
hungry between meals. There's nothing wrong with
snacking—as long as you choose healthy snacks.

If you're quitting smoking, snacks are a godsend in
more ways than one. Eating small and often stimulates
basic metabolism so you burn up more energy. Fat
people who leave most of their food until dinnertime
usually stay fat. Fat people who decide to eat meals
plus sensible snacks lose fat around the gut much more
effectively. It's not snacking itself that's the problem,
but the types of foods people use for snacks. As long

as you make wise choices of low-fat snacks, they should do no harm.

Good choices for snacks include:

- a slice of wholemeal bread wrapped round a banana
- a piece of fresh fruit—any type, including a wedge of melon, a punnet of strawberries or an apple, orange, pear, etc.
- a slice or two of raisin toast (use fat-reduced spread)
- a fresh bread roll (buy one fresh and eat it straight)
- air-popped popcorn (make at home, or buy when you are out, but ask for it to be served without butter)
- low-fat yoghurt (if flavoured, choose one without sugar)
- smoothie (blend some skim milk, a couple of ice cubes, a small banana and some sweetener, if desired)
- rye crackers with low-fat cheese and celery
- cup of soup
- frozen soft serve non-dairy fruit or fat-free yoghurt.

A sample daily food intake for waist loss

Although we are opposed to diets as such, the following gives an example of a good daily food intake for fat loss.

Breakfast
Wholegrain cereal, with low-fat milk, wholegrain bread, thin spread of reduced-fat butter or margarine, Vegemite, Marmite, honey or jam, tea/coffee.

Lunch
Sandwiches with fillings of lean meat and salad, plus fruit. Iced water. Use wholemeal bread. Fillings: salad with lean meat, lite cheese, canned tuna, chicken or turkey.

Dinner
Small portion of lean meat or chicken (no skin)
      or
Fish—large fillet
Large potato or rice/pasta
Large serve of vegetables/salad
Fruit
Tea/coffee (low-fat milk)

Snack
Low-fat yoghurt, bowl of cereal or bread

What about diets?

Some people are more suited to organised diet plans than others and some organised diet plans are better than others. Some diets are not recommended at all. They can be downright dangerous and *may make you fatter in the long run!*

Going 'on a diet' necessarily means coming off it at some stage and that means it can't be something that's done for life—so it won't work.

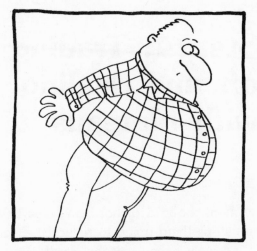

JACK DISCOVERS THE LEANING OF LIFE.

If you do like to be given some direction, and you are able to stick to a pre-planned diet and not be unduly influenced by outside temptations, an organised diet may be a useful approach, provided you think you can stick with it.

Some diets recommended for men are *The Super Pyramid Eating Program*; *Eat More, Weigh Less*; *The Pritikin Program*; *The Complete F-Plan Diet*; and *Weight Watchers Diet Plan—for Men*.

Not recommended are *Fit for Life*; *The Drinking Man's Diet*; *The Complete Scarsdale Medical Diet*; *Dr Atkins' Super Energy Diet*; *The 'Beverly Hills' Diet*; *The 'Grapefruit' Diet*; fasting; *The Zone Diet*; or any diet which promises fast weight loss. (For a detailed assessment of diet plans, check *The Diet Dilemma* by Rosemary Stanton (Allen & Unwin, Sydney, 1991).

8 Step 4: Trading off and dealing with plateaus

For many men, the idea of not being able to enjoy a drink often stops them trying to reduce their gut. And although, as we've seen, alcohol itself is not likely to be a cause of an enlarged waist, there are some other reasons why alcohol might be counter-productive. Alcohol may slow down the rate at which fat is burned in the body. And because it doesn't take much energy to convert fat in the blood to storage fat, the effects of alcohol with a fatty diet can mean that even more fat gets deposited on the belly. So, instead of fat in the diet being used as energy, it fills the fat cell reservoirs around the waist. If there was no fat in the diet, there would be negligible fat stored in the fat cells. But because it's almost impossible (and undesirable) to get rid of all the fat in the diet, there's likely to be some available for storage if there is a high alcohol intake. Also, it's easy to eat fatty foods (like chips and peanuts or cabanossi and crackers) with alcohol. You're much less likely to have an apple or a fruit salad with a beer!

If alcohol is consumed with sugary mixers (such as soft drink or fruit juice), the problem is made worse. The sugar in these, together with the alcohol, provides the body with enough calories, so any fat in the diet is sent for storage in the fat cells. Alcohol also decreases your inhibition and control. So while you may stoically refuse to even look at those crisps on the bar before you've had a drink, the more drinks you have, the more tempting they're likely to become.

There are also the compensatory effects of alcohol to consider. While you're drinking, you're not likely to be moving. And it's movement which burns up fat. Finally, for some reason which is still unclear, alcohol tends to increase a later craving for fatty foods. Have you noticed how you never crave a fresh salad sandwich after a night out? It's always something more greasy, like bacon and eggs. And it's these that cause the so-called beer gut.

Reasons why alcohol can make you fat

1 **Alcohol is generally eaten with fatty foods.**

2 Effects of added sugary mixers (e.g. soft drink, fruit juices).

3 Alcohol may slow fat metabolism.

4 Alcohol decreases inhibition and control and hence may lead to you eating and drinking more.

5 Movement levels are reduced while drinking.

6 Heavy drinking can lead to post-alcohol cravings.

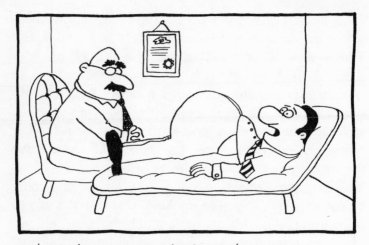

MILTON FINALLY SEEKS PSYCHIATRIC HELP IN AN EFFORT TO
UNDERSTAND HIS CONVICTION THAT A BEAR HAD CLIMBED
INTO HIS STOMACH TO HIBERNATE.

Fortunately, you don't have to give up all the good things in life. What's the point in making your life miserable? You can enjoy a drink *and* lose weight. But it means making some trade-offs. We'll look at these soon, but first let's see how much alcohol there is in different drinks and also look at why you may need to cut back.

Alcohol is defined in terms of a 'standard drink'. Western culture has been quite clever in working out different sizes of most drinks so they pack the same alcoholic punch. For example, the amounts of various drinks which have the equivalent of about 10 grams of alcohol are shown in the table below:

Standard drink sizes and types

Low-alcohol beer	2 × 285 mL (middie) (2 x 10 oz)	10 g alcohol
Ordinary beer	1 × 285 mL (middie)	10 g alcohol
Table wine	1 × 120 mL (4oz)	10 g alcohol
Fortified wine	1 × 60 mL (2oz)	10 g alcohol
Spirits	1 × 30mL (1oz)	10 g alcohol

Alcohol isn't the only component of a drink that determines its calorie content. Some drinks are also rich in sugar. As you can see from the table below, some drinks are higher in calories than others.

Energy content of various drinks

		Calories
Low-alcohol beer	285 mL middie (10 oz)	70
Regular beer	285 mL middie	105
Regular beer	370 mL can	140
Stout	285 mL middie	160
Table wine	125 mL (4 oz) glass	85
Fortified wine	60 mL (2 oz) glass	80
1 nip spirits	30 mL (1 oz) (with nothing added, except water or soda)	60
Orange juice	250 mL glass	90
Cola (sugared)	370 mL can	160
Orange-flavoured soft drink	370 mL can	200

This omits any mixers you may add. Fruit juices, cordial and soft drinks, for example, are even higher in calories than some alcoholic drinks. When they're added to alcohol (e.g. in brandy and dry, rum and cola, gin and tonic or champagne and orange juice), the calorie content is even higher.

Even within beers, there's a difference in calorie content. Some people ask if they should switch from beer to spirits. Beer contains a little more sugar than spirits, but this is so small that it's irrelevant. However, spirits are often consumed with sugary mixer drinks. Some people find they drink less when they switch to spirits; others drink more because the drinks are smaller and less filling. Stick with whichever you're able to drink in the least quantities. Wine is also a popular drink and some people wonder if it matters which wine they choose. From the point of view of calories, it makes very little difference. Sweeter wines have almost the same calorie value as dry wines.

To be able to enjoy a drink and lose weight, you'll need to make some trade-offs in the type of food you eat and the amount of exercise you do. As a rough guide, one *10 ounce* glass of beer is fairly equivalent to walking or jogging 1.5 kilometres (about a mile), although the effect of exercise on metabolic rate may reduce this distance slightly. Alternatively, a *10 ounce* glass of beer is equivalent to a couple of biscuits or a small piece of cake. To balance out up to 4 beers a day, you can decrease the amount of biscuits, cake or equivalent fatty food you eat, or increase your walking. The chart below gives you an idea of with what and to what degree you can make trade-offs.

The beer drinker's 'trade-off' guide

If you drink ...	you *must* (daily)	you *should* also
1 alcoholic drink a day (1 middie beer or 1 nip spirits with diet mixers)	• eat low-fat foods • reduce soft drinks and fruit juices to between one and two a day	• walk ten minutes a day and walk instead of drive or ride
2 alcoholic drinks a day	do all the above PLUS: • cut out cakes/biscuits with morning or afternoon tea • eat more fruit/vegetables • remove chicken skin and cut all fat off meat • stop adding sugar—you can use sugar substitutes	• walk twenty minutes a day • reduce fried foods and size of meat serve • eat more fish
3–4 alcoholic drinks a day*	do all the above PLUS: • not skip meals and never miss breakfast • eat a light salad lunch • reduce meat/protein foods in all meals • avoid sweets or substitute fruit, and never eat after dinner	• walk (or do other aerobic exercise) for 40 minutes a day • walk up stairs (don't use escalators) • change the TV channels manually • don't ask the kids to get things—get them yourself!

If you drink ...	**you *must* (daily)**	**you *should* also**
3–4 alcoholic drinks a day*	• use spreads (butter/margarine) thinly	• have two AFDs (alcohol free days) each week

* World Health Organisation authorities warn that more than 4 alcoholic drinks a day can be a health risk. Three drinks in an hour can also raise blood alcohol above levels safe for driving for men. Women's blood alcohol levels will be too high for safe driving at even lower levels and alcohol is also a strong risk factor for breast cancer in women.

Soft drinks and fruit juices

Many working men who want to lose weight fall into the trap of cutting back on grog and drinking soft drinks, such as cola drinks, instead. Some men even skip breakfast or lunch to try to lose weight. In our experience, it's not uncommon for such men to have up to ten—or even twenty—bottles of coke in a day!

Soft drink is often more of a problem to many men wanting to lose weight than beer or alcohol.

Most people also think of fruit juices as being healthy—which they are, because they have more vitamins than soft drink. But fruit is high in fruit sugars, and when juice is separated from the fibre of its fruit, the bulk is reduced and it becomes easy to take in all the sugar and calories from three to four pieces of fruit in one drink. It might be fine for someone who's not fat, but it's not much use to anyone trying to solve a waist problem.

There's no real need for fruit juices. The hype that says you must have orange juice for breakfast is a bit of a con job. It's better to eat a few pieces of fruit (say, three to four a day) and get your fibre intake up. Fruit cordials are even worse because they have concentrated sugar in place of most of the nutrients of the fruit.

The obvious solution is to cut back on, or cut out, regular soft drinks, fruit juices and cordials. The best alternative is water or mineral water as they have no calories. If you can't stomach these and you really want a sweet drink, diet drinks are the next best choice. They also have no calories, although some researchers have found that their artificial sweeteners might increase appetite so you later eat more than you've saved by having low-energy drinks. Those who don't find these drinks increase their appetite may find them useful.

Fat is a great insulator, so an overweight man gets hot easily. When this happens, you sweat, and then you need to replace the lost fluid. If you replace fluids with alcoholic drinks, soft drinks or fruit juice, you'll take in lots of energy. If you've still got a high fat content in your daily food intake, you'll get fatter, sweat more, drink more of these drinks and continue in a vicious cycle. Alcohol is also a diuretic, so it makes you lose more fluid in urine than the drink provides. Far from rehydrating the body, alcohol causes dehydration, as you'll know from the amount of time you spend at the urinal in any pub. If you're going to drink

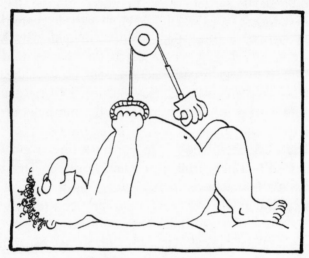

TECHNO-EROTICISM

alcohol, always drink water first, especially if you've been sweating heavily. Water is not a diuretic like alcohol and it's not high in sugar like fruit juices or cordials.

Drinks intake questionnaire

1 How often do you drink alcohol? (circle a number)

Every day	4
4–5 days a week	3
2–3 days a week	2
1–2 days a week	1
Never drink alcohol	1

2   When you drink alcohol how much do you usually drink (1 standard drink is a middie of beer, 1 nip of spirits or 1 glass of wine)?

More than 10 drinks	4
5–10 drinks	3
2–4 drinks	2
1–2 drinks	1
Never drink alcohol	0

3   How often do you drink soft drinks? (don't count diet drinks)

Every day	4
4–5 days a week	3
2–3 days a week	2
1–2 days a week	1
Never drink soft drinks	0

4   When you drink soft drinks (not counting diet drinks) how much do you usually drink?

More than 10 drinks	4
5–10 drinks	3
2–4 drinks	2
1–2 drinks	1
Never drink soft drinks	0

5   How often do you drink fruit juices?

Every day	4
4–5 days a week	3
2–3 days a week	2
1–2 days a week	1
Never drink fruit juices	0

6   When you drink fruit juices how much do you usually drink?

More than 10 drinks   4
5–10 drinks   3
2–4 drinks   2
1–2 drinks   1
Never drink fruit juices   0

Scores: Multiply questions 1 × 2; 3 × 4; and 5 × 6. If you scored 1 or less than 1 on any combination, your weight doesn't seem to be influenced by your drink intake.

If you scored between 1 and 4 on any combination your weight might be influenced by either alcohol (Q1 × 2), soft drink (Q3 × 4) or fruit juice (Q4 × 5).

If you scored more than 4 on any combination, your weight will definitely be influenced by either alcohol (Q1 × 2), soft drink (Q3 × 4) or fruit juice (Q4 × 5).

Having said all that, we also suggest that if you're a drinker and you intend to make the most of the GutBuster program, you must *not* go off the grog (unless of course you really want to). You're unlikely to stay abstemious for the rest of your life, and in line with the principles of this program, to lose your gut successfully you need to make permanent changes. Once you come back to drinking, everything else you do will go out the window. So it's important that you learn to live with and enjoy your drink. For that reason, it's also encouraging to know that it's not the alcohol, but the food that goes with it, that's likely to make you fat.

For general good health, everyone should drink plenty of water. When you eat more fibre, you should also drink more water. If you can't bear to drink water in public, do it in private—but make sure you have enough. Most people need about 8 standard-size (250 mL) glasses of water a day. You may need much more in summer, or if your work or exercise makes you sweat a lot. You should drink enough water so that your urine is clear by mid-morning. If it's yellow, you're not drinking enough.

What about coffee or tea? These have practically no calories, so they're unlikely to make you fat from excess calories unless you're adding lots of milk or sugar. The caffeine content may even act as a stimulant and help to reduce appetite. But, as we pointed out earlier, caffeine in large doses can increase nervousness and anxiety and you can have withdrawal symptoms if you don't maintain your regular dose. The body can also become habituated to caffeine, and small doses will fail to act as a stimulant if you regularly have large doses. Up to three or four cups of coffee a day are unlikely to cause harm and may be helpful. Any more may have limited or even negative effects.

In summary, you *can* enjoy a drink and lose fat at the same time. The answer is in balancing the extra energy intake (particularly reducing soft drinks) with extra energy output, such as walking. If this is combined with a good, sensible, low-fat, high-fibre diet, it won't take you long to become a 'GutBuster'.

Plateauing and what to do about it

If you've been on any weight loss program, and you've lost weight, it's inevitable that you'll reach a plateau at some stage when nothing more seems to happen. This is perfectly natural. It's nature's way of stopping you from disappearing. Many people, especially women, will give up at this stage, thinking that nothing's working, In fact, your body wouldn't be working properly if you *didn't* reach a plateau. It may happen after a week. It may be a month, it may be six months. But one thing's for sure: unless you only have a little fat to lose, you'll plateau at least once, and possibly several times over several months or years, before you get down to your goal waist size.

If you look at the graph below, you'll see what this means. Most diet programs assume that you'll keep losing weight in a continual fashion as shown in the straight line in the graph. Of course this is not so. Unless you've only got a little to lose, you'll come down in stages as shown by the bent line in the graph. The longer you've carried the extra weight, the more likely it is that the decreases will be smaller and the plateaus

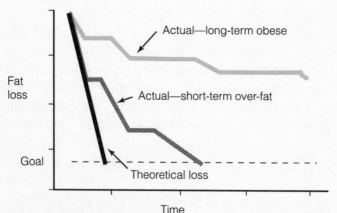

Figure 7: Plateaus in fat loss

longer. Also, the more you lose, the smaller the drops and the longer the plateaus will be. This is your body defending itself against the possibility of starvation.

The key to success in any long-term fat-loss program is to understand that while you're on a plateau you're winning! It's only if you start to put on weight that you begin to lose again. The more gradually you lose, the less likely you are to plateau and the less likely you are to bounce back fatter than ever. So don't be disillusioned with a gradual but steady waist loss.

If you understand what a plateau is, you should be able to work out how to get off it and continue losing. A plateau is a period of adjustment where your body has become used to your new lifestyle. It has adapted to the walking you're doing and is now able to do it more easily. For that reason, you're using less energy than when you first started and hence less fat is burned. Because you've probably also lost some weight, it costs you less energy to walk the same distance compared with when you were heavier. You also eat less food because you don't need as much as you did for a big body. Body fat levels are designed to reach a plateau so that you won't keep losing weight to the point of death.

To get off a plateau, you need to do something to oppose the body's adaptation. And what you need is change. Try changing the type and amount of food you eat, or the type, frequency, intensity or duration of the exercise you do. If you've spent your time walking, try swimming or cycling just to unblock the system. If you've been eating only English food, try some Mongolian or Lithuanian (low-fat of course). Once you've

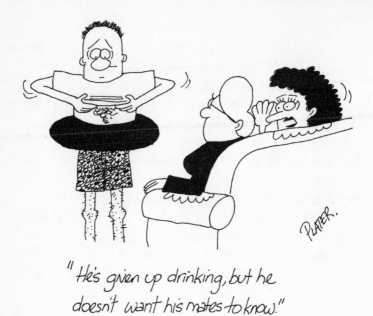

"He's given up drinking, but he doesn't want his mates to know."

broken through a plateau, you may go back to doing what you were doing before. But remember, make sure it's something you can do for life.

Appendix 1: What happens when we get fat? Some basic physiology

Fat, is stored in special fat cells (called adipocytes) that exist throughout the body, but in biggest numbers around the mid-section of men, and the thighs, buttocks and breasts of women. A fat cell is pretty much like any other body cell except that it contains a little pool of fat, or a fat store, called a lipid (fat) pool. It looks a bit like that shown in Figure A1.

Fat cells are scattered throughout most of the body—in muscle, in bone, around organs, under the skin. About the only places where there are no fat cells are the eyelids, part of the cranium or skull, the lungs and—perhaps surprisingly—the penis and scrotum of men.

Although it gets a bit complicated, it's useful to understand the basics of how fat is stored in, and taken from, fat cells. If you know about this, it makes it easier to understand the proper ways to reduce fat, and why

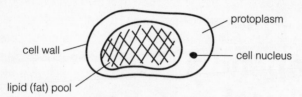

Figure A1:   Representation of a fat cell

some of the traditional approaches to weight control not only don't work, but can actually make you fatter!

How fat cells work

There's only a couple of things you need to know about fat cells to understand how (and why) they work. Fat cells collect and store fat when there's an over-supply of energy from what we eat and drink. They also release this fat when it's needed to be burned as energy in the muscles.

Think of fat cells as being like a lot of little water bags that fill up and expand when there's plenty of rain, and empty out and shrink in prolonged periods of drought. The part that expands and contracts in the fat cell is the lipid, or fat pool, which is a reservoir of fats known as triglycerides. These can take up to 95 per cent of the fat cell. The effect is shown in Figure A2.

What makes these fat cells do these things? Let's look first at how the fat cells fill up.

The excess 'water' or 'rain' that we're talking about in the water bag case is food floating around in the bloodstream in the case of fat cells. It can be in the

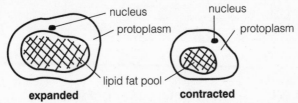

Figure A2: Expanded and contracted fat cells

form of fat from fatty foods, but it can also be in the form of glucose, or sugars that come more directly from carbohydrates in foods. This food 'energy' in the bloodstream can be either burned up in the muscle, like fuel in an engine, which makes the muscle contract allowing us to move, or it will look for a home until it's needed as fuel at a time when not enough extra fuel (food) is coming in, or when too much is being used up in exercise.

The body, like an engine, is fussy about the type of fuel it prefers. It always prefers to burn glucose rather than fat. To break fat down to the form in which it can be used in the muscle takes much more effort and, unlike glucose, it needs to have oxygen present to do this. It's a bit like comparing paper and wood as fuels in a fire.

So glucose (from carbohydrate-rich foods like cereals, pasta, fruit and vegetables) is used up directly from the bloodstream. If there's more carbohydrate than is needed, it is housed in either the liver or the muscle itself, for quick access when it's required. In the unlikely situation that there's still more than is needed, it's then shunted into the fat cells and turned into fat to be kept

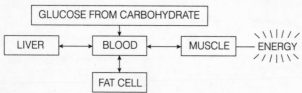

Figure A3:   Carbohydrate and fat storage

there in longer term storage. This process is shown in Figure A3.

Glucose, however, is a rather large-sized chemical molecule. On its own, it has difficulty getting from the bloodstream through the walls of ordinary cells like fat or muscle cells. So it has a helper. *Insulin* is a hormone (or a chemical 'trigger') produced by the pancreas. It acts as a 'gate-keeper' for blood glucose, making it able to pass through the cell wall and into the cell more easily. The amount of insulin produced is related to the amount of glucose taken into the bloodstream after a meal. In some conditions (e.g. diabetes), the body produces less insulin, or the insulin it produces becomes less effective, and the glucose never reaches the cells, starving them of energy and, if the condition is left untreated, eventually killing the individual. The impact of insulin is shown in Figure A4.

As we'll see, the role of insulin is an important one for the person worried about being overweight because not only does it help increase body fat if the situation is right, but if there's too much fat, this can cause a problem in insulin production and wind up leading to diabetes. This will become clearer as we go along. But first, let's look at the role of fat.

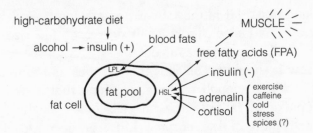

Figure A4: Influences on fat cell metabolism

Large amounts of fat in the bloodstream are only likely to be used up directly as energy (in any significant amount) if the body's supplies of glucose have run out. Otherwise, fat is acted upon by an enzyme (or chemical which speeds up a reaction), called LPL (lipoprotein lipase) to make it into the type of fats (triglycerides) which can be stored away in the most readily available fat cells. This process is called 'lipogenesis' (the making of fat). It expands the size of the fat cells it fills up.

If the body keeps taking in too much food and not burning up enough energy, these fat cells will continue to get bigger. If, on the other hand, less food comes in, or more fuel is needed as more energy is expended, fat in the fat cells will be called on to be reconverted back to fatty acids in the bloodstream and then broken down into a form which can be used like glucose in the muscle.

This breakdown of fats in the fat cells and transmission back into the bloodstream is carried out by another enzyme, called HSL (or hormone sensitive lipase), which exists in the fat cell. The process of breaking down fat in the fat cell and making it available as energy is called 'lipolysis'. It decreases the size of the fat cell as it empties it out.

Now it should be obvious that, as well as too much food and not enough exercise, anything that increases the uptake of fat into the fat cells—such as through the activation of the enzyme LPL—or decreases the breakdown of fat such as through the deactivation of the enzyme HSL, will result in an increase in body fat. On the other hand, anything that does the opposite will decrease fat. The big question is, can this be done?

There are a number of factors known, and suspected to have this effect. These are shown in Figure A4. Let's look at these independently.

The role of insulin

As we've seen, one factor known to influence fat building is the hormone insulin. It's now known, for example, that insulin increases the action of LPL in fat cells and suppresses the action of HSL. This would increase the rate at which fat is stored because, while more is being stored, less is being broken down. So anything that increases insulin when there's fat or glucose that's not being used as energy floating around in the blood is likely to increase the build-up of fat in the cell.

Insulin, of course, is increased by glucose in the bloodstream. The two act in partnership. So if glucose is present in high quantities when fat is present, it's more likely that fat will be stored in fat cells. In simple terms, this suggests that if a high-sugar meal is eaten in conjunction with a high-fat meal the fat in the food is more likely to become fat on you than if the meal was either high-sugar or high-fat alone.

That this is true has now been reasonably well documented. Not only have the biochemical effects been shown, but it's been found that if animals that are given meals of high fat and sugar together (typical of most processed 'sweet foods' you buy), they get greater increases in fat stores than if either is taken separately. Interestingly, it's this fat–sweet combination which also seems to be attractive—it can actually give you a craving for what you may think is 'sweet' food, but is in fact sweet/fat food. The old idea of a 'sweet tooth' is not exactly accurate: it's just as much a 'fat tooth'.

The lesson from this is that not only should fatty foods be reduced in the diet for fat loss, but that fatty *and* sweet foods (like chocolate, cake and biscuits) might be best avoided more than either fatty foods alone (e.g. chips) or sweet foods alone (e.g. meringue, lollies). About the worst example of a meal for losing weight, if this is true, would be a fatty main course followed by a dessert high in sugar.

Another way of increasing blood insulin is with alcohol. Being high in sugar, alcohol also enhances fat deposits in fat cells. And because the fat cells most willing to be filled up in men are those around the stomach, it stands to reason that big drinkers who also eat high-fat diets often wind up with what's known as a 'beer gut'. Alcohol, then, is best accompanied by a low-fat meal, rather than the traditional high-fat foods (e.g. pies, chips) that so often seem to go with it.

Enhancing HSL

On the other side of the equation, we've said that things which enhance the activity of HSL would speed up the breakdown of fat from fat cells. The chemicals best known for doing this are the hormones adrenalin and cortisol, both of which are produced in reaction to stress, either physical or emotional. They can also be influenced by stimulant drugs (like the amphetamines that are often used as appetite suppressants) and may even be affected by common stimulants like caffeine.

Most important amongst these, though, is physical activity, because this increases the rate of fat breakdown, and uses up the resultant free fatty acids (FFAs) to power the muscles for movement. Emotional stress, on the other hand, while it may do the former, doesn't do the latter, because the body isn't necessarily moving any more. Hence a mass of fat is left to circulate in the bloodstream with nowhere to go and with the potential of 'clogging up' the arteries and causing a thrombosis or a heart attack. The best type of exercise for avoiding the effects of stress is gentle continuous exercise because, as explained above, fat needs oxygen to be burned in muscle. Anaerobic exercise (without 'air', or oxygen), which is short sharp bursts of physical activity, doesn't use oxygen and therefore doesn't have the same effect.

Metabolism and fat deposition

For food and energy to be shifted around the body, used up in muscle, or for it to supply energy to essential organs or be deposited in fat cells requires effort on behalf of the body. This is an ongoing process. In fact, the body uses up about one Calorie (4.2 kJ) per minute, just to keep everything running well enough to stay alive. Both of the processes referred to above (e.g. building up and breaking down fat in fat cells) require energy, so activities that influence them will increase the metabolic rate.

Eating increases metabolic rate for a short time after a meal or a snack because energy is required to digest the food, distribute nutrients round the body and burn them as energy or store them as fat. The process of digestion gives off energy as heat, and this is called the 'thermic effect' of food. (You may have noticed how you warm up on a cold day after eating.) Exercise also has the same effect probably over a longer period, because it requires energy to break down fuels and make them available in the form required by the muscles and then to replenish the muscles after the exercise has been completed.

Again, in practical terms, the implications of this are that small (low-fat) meals eaten several times a day will have a greater fat-burning effect than one large meal only. If, as is usually the case with dieting men, this large meal is eaten just before retiring (when the metabolic rate slows down), and if it consists of a high-fat main course and sweets for 'afters', accompanied by the odd drop of alcohol, the recipe for a fat gut is well in the making.

Types of fat cells

Now we've seen *how* fat cells expand and contract, it's also of interest to see *where* they do this most easily. Men know, for example, that they generally put on fat first around the waist. But women—at least those in their early years—put it on the breasts and the backs of the arms, but most commonly on the hips and buttocks. (After menopause, women take on the added fat cells characteristic of men—that is, around the stomach, probably due to the decrease in activity of female hormones.)

Although fat cells everywhere are basically the same, there are some differences in the way they function. It's known, for example, that the fat cells around the hips and buttocks of women are smaller and less 'lypolytic' (i.e. they give up their fat stores less easily) than those on the breasts and upper body or around the waists of men (see Figure A5).

One reason for this may be greater activity of LPL, or 'fat-building' enzymes, and the decreased activity of HSL or 'fat-breaking-down' enzymes which has commonly been found in and around fat cells on the hips and buttocks of women, compared with those on the upper body and on men. It's not yet known why this is the case, but it appears to be related to the male and female hormones, particularly testosterone (in men) and oestrogen (in women). It's known, for example, that males on oestrogen treatment (for various medical

Figure A5:   Male/female fat cell deposition

problems) tend to put on weight around the hips and buttocks. Females who lose the benefits of oestrogen on the other hand (i.e. after menopause), tend to take on a more masculine shape.

From an evolutionary viewpoint, the resistance of lower body fat cells is significant, because it allows greater storage of energy (fat) to enable a woman to survive through the nine months of pregnancy and when breastfeeding, in case there's a shortage of food. The larger and more lypolytic fat cells around the waists of men appear to have no such constraint to their breakdown of fat. In fact, they're usually the first place from which fat disappears when a man changes his energy balance. It's thought that this may have developed evolutionary significance to act as an immediate energy store for hunter-gatherers to save 'fuel' in the good times to help them through the lean times. However, the consequences of this over the long term are much more severe than for the excess fat stored around the hips and buttocks of women. As we've shown, there is a risk of thrombosis and heart disease from too much fat clogging up the arteries. An excess of this type of fat around the middle can also cause cells to develop 'insulin resistance' and this can lead to the development of diabetes—a disease which, in its adult form, is highly associated with being overweight.

Upper and lower body obesity is determined by the waist-to-hip ratio measure described in Chapter 3. For the reasons outlined above, upper body obesity is more of a threat to good health than lower body obesity and hence males (and post-menopausal females) are most likely to be at risk.

Appendix 2: Alcohol and fat

Alcohol and metabolism

Alcohol is basically a toxin (poison) to the body, and the body has several ways of disposing of it as quickly as possible. These involve enzymes, including:

- gastric alcohol dehydrogenase enzyme (ADH)
- alcohol dehydrogenase enzyme (ADH) produced in the liver in several forms
- catalase-hydrogen peroxide system.

As the third option accounts for less than 2 per cent of ethanol removal, we won't discuss it here.

Alcohol dehydrogenase

The production of gastric alcohol dehydrogenase metabolises about 30 per cent of the ethanol consumed by men and 10 per cent of that consumed by women. This enzyme is less active in those who abuse alcohol and also declines with age.

Within the liver, alcohol dehydrogenase metabolises moderate quantities of alcohol. A second hepatic (liver) enzyme comes into play with moderate to high, or excessive, alcohol intake.

Each of the liver enzymes that metabolises alcohol produce a substance called acetaldehyde, which is then metabolised further to acetate and acetyl-CoA. However, the reactions of the two liver enzymes have different effects and different consequences from the nutritional viewpoint.

If you're interested in biochemistry, you may like to know that while oxidising ethanol, gastric alcohol dehydrogenase suppresses the citric acid cycle, preferentially producing lactate from pyruvate, reducing gluconeogenesis and lowering excretion of uric acid. The potential results of these reactions are acidosis, low levels of blood glucose and high levels of uric acid. More fatty acids are also synthesised and very low-density lipoproteins (VLDL) and high-density lipoproteins (HDL) increase. Reduced oxidation of fatty acids increases the oxidation of ethanol, increasing production of adenosine triphosphate (ATP).

The second hepatic enzyme (produced when higher quantities of alcohol are consumed) does not generate ATP and does not lead to synthesis of body fat. With this system, as ethanol is oxidised to acetaldehyde, fatty acid oxidation is inhibited. The result may be fatty liver. While this reaction is occurring, increased quantities of catecholamines are released. These favour peripheral lipolysis and ketoacidosis, and reduce the activity of antioxidants produced in the body. This can lead to liver damage, especially if the diet is high in fat.

Polyunsaturated fats are an extra potential problem in these circumstances, because they increase the body's requirements for antioxidants. This system is energy wasteful, increases metabolic rate by 7–10 per cent and wastes kilojoules. It also increases degradation of protein and thus reduces lean body mass—an effect which can be seen in people with alcoholism.

In those who habitually consume moderate–high levels of alcohol, much of the energy from alcohol is wasted. This has been observed in many studies showing that by adding 90 grams of ethanol a day (the equivalent of a 750 mL bottle of wine or nine 250 mL glasses of beer) male volunteers lost weight, even though their total calories were maintained at their normal level. Studies also show that adding alcohol to a single meal inhibits fat oxidation, with a somewhat lesser effect on carbohydrate oxidation. This is due to the dissipation of energy during metabolism of ethanol.

If you consume fat and alcohol together, the liver does not oxidise fats and they can accumulate in liver cells. Because of this, we have concentrated on reducing fat in the diet rather than removing alcohol. However, we do not promote excessive consumption of alcohol and believe that overall intake should be less than that currently consumed by many men. By moderating alcohol, rather than cutting it out, and also restricting fat, we believe many men may find it easier to adopt changes they can live with.

Alcohol can also inhibit lipoprotein lipase, an enzyme that splits triglycerides and leads to uptake of fatty acids as adipose tissue and muscle. Alcohol suppresses the activity of this enzyme, which means that the liver is exposed to higher levels of triglycerides.

Lower rates of fat oxidation and increased synthesis of triglycerides lead to increased storage of fat in the liver.

As well as the biochemical effect of ethanol metabolism within the body, there is plenty of epidemiological evidence showing that alcohol is not converted into body fat. On the contrary, several studies show an inverse association, especially in women. It is possible that this is due to drinkers eating less, although alcohol contributes 7 Calories per gram and overall caloric intake does not appear to be lower. Clinical studies dating from the early 1980s show that substituting an equal number of calories from alcohol for calories from food results in less weight gain in drinkers. Several reviews emphasise these findings.

Alcohol does participate in the energy cycle, although less so in heavy drinkers since they metabolise alcohol through an enzyme system with much more energy wastage. Alcohol can also increase the rate of fat synthesis, but does this much more in rodents than in humans, where the rate is very slow. The most important effect of alcohol is that it floods the liver with fat and increases synthesis of triglycerides. So, if dietary fat or total caloric intake is high, this easily leads to fatty liver—an undesirable condition and one to be avoided.

The message about alcohol is this: moderate consumption (less than four drinks a day for men and one or two for women) combined with a low-fat diet fits in with waist loss.

Appendix 3:
The Exerselector
Questionnaire

The exerselector questionnaire

Instructions

1 Circle the number under each exercise corresponding to the answer in each category. Add scores down the column for each exercise to get your TOTAL TEST SCORES.

	Walking/jogging	Dancing	Weight training	Circuit training	Mini-trampolining	Aerobics to music	Swimming	Skipping/stepping	Cycling	Ball games
Personal details										
Age:										
Under 35	0	0	0	0	5	0	0	0	0	0
35–49	0	1	0	0	5	0	0	3	0	4
50–59	2	3	1	1	1	3	0	5	3	5
60+	4	4	9	4	0	7	0	8	7	6
Body frame:										
Small/medium	0	0	0	0	0	0	0	0	0	0
Large	3	2	0	1	0	1	0	4	0	2
Are you										
. . . more than a little overweight?										
No	0	0	0	0	0	0	0	0	0	0
Yes	4	4	0	3	0	4	0	5	3	6
. . . an indoor or outdoor type of person?										
Indoor	7	0	0	0	0	0	4	0	6	4

	Walking/jogging	Dancing	Weight training	Circuit training	Mini-trampolining	Aerobics to music	Swimming	Skipping/stepping	Cycling	Ball games
Outdoor	0	0	1	1	5	1	2	5	1	0
... self-conscious about exercising in public?										
No	0	0	0	0	0	0	0	0	0	0
Yes	5	7	3	0	0	8	4	0	4	5
... competitive?										
very	3	8	1	2	4	1	3	8	5	0
moderately	0	5	0	1	3	1	3	5	4	2
not very	0	0	0	0	0	0	3	0	2	8
... prepared to pay more than $10 a week to exercise?										
Yes	0	0	0	0	0	0	0	0	0	0
No	0	4	8	0	1	8	1	0	2	4
... suffering limiting injuries to any of the following?										
Legs/ankles/knees	9	7	1	5	3	9	1	9	4	7
shoulders/arms	1	2	6	4	0	7	3	4	2	5
hip	9	7	1	3	3	9	3	8	3	7
back	5	6	2	4	1	10	2	5	5	6
... NOT within easy access (say 15 mins) of any of the following?										
pool/lake/sea	0	0	0	0	0	0	10	0	0	0
park/open space	5	0	0	0	0	0	0	0	0	0
gymnasium	0	3	9	0	0	5	0	0	0	4

	Walking/ jogging	Dancing	Weight training	Circuit training	Mini- trampolining	Aerobics to music	Swimming	Skipping/ stepping	Cycling	Ball games
sports facilities	0	0	0	0	0	0	0	0	0	10
safe bike routes	0	0	0	0	0	0	0	0	10	0
... prepared to give up daily time 3–4 days a week?										
less than 20 mins	4	10	5	3	3	9	10	3	5	10
20–40 mins	0	2	0	0	0	2	4	0	1	4
more than 40 mins	0	0	0	0	0	0	0	0	0	0
... a person who prefers										
exercising alone	0	5	0	1	0	10	0	0	0	0
exercising with a friend	1	0	0	1	6	9	2	3	2	0
exercising in a group	2	0	8	1	10	0	2	6	4	0

Total test scores

	—	—	—	—	—	—	—	—	—	—

2 Calculate your INTEREST SCORE for each activity.

If you think you'd enjoy carrying out the activity regularly, give yourself an INTEREST SCORE of 100.

If you think you may enjoy carrying out the activity regularly, give yourself an INTEREST SCORE of 90.

If the activity doesn't appeal give yourself an INTEREST SCORE of 80.

Interest score

———

3 Calculate a FINAL SCORE for each activity by subtracting the TOTAL TEST SCORE from the INTEREST SCORE for each activity.

Final score

___

4   The activity with the highest FINALSCORE will generally be the most appropriate aerobic exercise for you. If there are several activities at the top falling within about 5 points of each other, choose the one you think you would prefer, or combine them as part of the one program.

Exerselector score sheet

Write your FINAL SCORES for each exercise in the appropriate position and then rank these from highest to lowest. In the position marked most appropriate exercise(s), write that exercise ranked number 1 and any other exercise within 10 points on FINAL SCORE from that exercise. This (or these) exercise(s), is (are) the one(s) selected as most appropriate for you.

Aerobic activity	**Final score**	**Ranking**
Walking, jogging	_____	_____
Swimming	_____	
Cycling	_____	
Ball games	_____	
Dancing	_____	
Skipping, stepping	_____	
Aerobics to music	_____	
Weight training	_____	
Circuit training	_____	
Mini-trampolining	_____	

YOUR CHOSEN EXERCISE(S)

1 _____
2 _____
3 _____
4 _____

Motivation

Your FINAL SCORE for your chosen exercise also tells you something about your level of motivation.

If your FINAL SCORE was **90 or more**, your motivation is high. You should have no trouble with your exercise program.

If your FINAL SCORE was **between 80 and 90**, your motivation is only average. You may need someone to help push you along, at least in the early stages.

If your FINAL SCORE was **less than 80**, your motivation is low. You'll definitely need someone to push you along, particularly in the early stages until you are fit enough to enjoy your chosen exercise, not for what it does for you but for itself.

Further reading

Egger, G. *Trim for Life*, Allen & Unwin, Sydney, 1997.

Egger G. and Champion, N. *The Fitness Leader's Handbook*, 4th edn. Kangaroo Press, Sydney, 1998.

Egger, G. and Stanton, R. *GutBuster 2: The High Energy Guide*, Allen & Unwin, Sydney, 1995.

Egger, G. and Swinburn, B. *The Fat Loss Handbook: A guide for Professionals*, Allen & Unwin, Sydney, 1996.

Stanton, R. *Eating for Peak Performance*, Allen & Unwin, Sydney, 1989.

Stanton, R. *The Diet Dilemma*, Allen & Unwin, Sydney, 1991.

Stanton, R. *Rosemary Stanton's Fat and Fibre Counter,* Wilkinson Books, Melbourne, 1993.

Stanton, R. *GutBuster Recipes*, Allen & Unwin, Sydney, 1994.

Stanton, R. *Good Fats. Bad Fats*, Allen & Unwin, Sydney, 1997.

Tuppling, H. *A Weight off Your Mind*, Allen & Unwin, Sydney, 1988.

Other books by these authors

Garry Egger

The art of sensible exercise
The fitness leader's exercise bible
The sport drug
Commonsense health
Fitness in six weeks
The Australian home fitness test
Running high
The fat loss handbook
Health promotion strategies and methods
Health and media
Trim for life

Rosemary Stanton

The diet dilemma
Eating for peak performance
Rosemary Stanton's healthy cooking
Food for under 5s
Food for health
Food and you
*Rosemary Stanton's complete book
  of food and nutrition*
Find out about fibre
Good fats, bad fats
Healthy vegetarian eating
Windbreaks

GUTBUSTER RECIPES

The companion to the GutBuster Waist Loss Guide

Rosemary Stanton

Over 100 recipes designed for men who want

- food that is good-tasting
- food that's filling
- food that will help them lose their waists
- food that's easy to prepare

No previous cooking experience is needed to make these tasty and satisfying soups, barbecues, stir-fries, pasta and rice dishes, salads, vegetables and delicious desserts. Rosemary Stanton has devised recipes that are fast and easy to prepare, and will produce results that will have your friends and family clamouring for more—without knowing they are eating low-fat food!

ISBN 1 86373 703 0

THE HIGH ENERGY GUIDE: GUTBUSTER 2

Garry Egger & Rosemary Stanton

On average, men die six years earlier than women, suffer twice the rate of heart disease and one-and-a-half times the rate of respiratory disease. But you can defy these statistics.

The GutBuster Waist Loss Guide gave you a simple 4-step approach to waist loss. *The High Energy Guide* looks at other factors which may not at first seem directly related to fat loss: new aspects of nutrition and exercise; behaviour changes and ways to keep you motivated; how to control stress; and how to recognise and prevent the major diseases associated with fatness and middle age.

So increase your odds for a long and healthy life and join the thousands of men busting a gut to change those statistics!

ISBN 1 86373 900 9